DATE DUE

Hospitals
& Patients

Hospitals & Patients

William R. Rosengren

Mark Lefton

AldineTransaction
A Division of Transaction Publishers
New Brunswick (U.S.A.) and London (U.K.)

Second paperback printing 2009
Copyright © 1969 by Transaction Publishers.

This book is printed on acid-free paper that meets the American National Standard for Permanence of Paper for Printed Library Materials.

Library of Congress Catalog Number: 2007015194
ISBN: 978-0-202-30947-7
Printed in the United States of America

Library of Congress Cataloging-in-Publication Data

Rosengren, William R., 1929-
    Hospitals and patients / William R. Rosengren and Mark Lefton.
        p. cm.
    Originally published: New York : Atherton Press, 1969.
    Includes bibliographical references and index.
    ISBN-13: 978-0-202-30947-7 (alk. paper)
    1. Hospitals—United States. 2. Medical care—United States. I. Lefton, Mark. II. Title.
    [DNLM: 1. Hospitals—trends—United States. 2. Hospital Administration—-United States. 3. Hospital—Patient Relations—United States. 4. Hospitalization—United States. 5. Sociology, Medical—United States. WX 100 R82E 1969a]

RA980.R67   2007
362.11—dc22   2007015194

Contents

PART III

Preface and Acknowledgments

This preface is deliberately brief in the hope that this will encourage its being read.

We try to accomplish four tasks in this book and to relate them one to the other. The first is to draw together, in a relatively small space, a summary of the sociological literature dealing with the structure and operation of hospitals of all kinds. Second, attention is drawn to the many newer ways of delivering medical services, most of which have received only passing attention by sociologists. Third, we try to organize these materials in terms of prevailing models for organizational analysis used by sociologists in studying and explaining what occurs in hospitals. Finally, we set forth an analytic model of organizations in the hope that it may be useful in drawing together seemingly divergent findings concerning hospitals, as well as in yielding some understanding of the "new" as well as the "old" forms of medical organization.

As a result of focusing upon the hospital, we have not referred to a good deal of research in medical sociology. Absent are the many studies of the doctor-patient relationship, determinants of sick-role behavior, epidemiological studies of both functional and organic illnesses, and others. We have selected those materials which in our judgment bear most directly upon relationships between the *patient as a person and the hospital as an organizational system.* Hence, this book does not purport to review the literature in medical sociology, only that part of it preoccupied with transactions between the person and the organization.

Part I highlights the importance of illness and hospitalization, and draws initial attention to the several ways in which the traditional hospital system has given way to more novel forms of medical organization. The intention here is to underscore the considerable gap between what have heretofore stood as serviceable frames of reference for the study of hospitals and what is actually occurring in the field of medical organization.

Part II is divided into three chapters. The first deals with the hospital as an organizational entity in both its bureaucratic and social-system aspects. The second treats processes of social interaction as they have been found to take place within the walls of medical institutions. The third deals with relationships between hospitals and their environments—community settings, larger institutional systems, and other *medically* relevant organizations. Finally, attention is turned to the different ways in which hospitals may elect to define their "patient materials" and the consequences this may have for structural arrangements to contend with these definitions, interpersonal relationships in hospitals, and linkages with other medical organizations.

Part III also contains three chapters—corresponding in perspective to those in Part II—the hospital as an organization; the patient *in* the hospital; and inter-hospital relationships. The integrating theme in these three chapters is contained in the client biography model.

This perspective stems from the proposition that a distinctive feature of people-processing organizations such as hospitals is that they interrupt the present and future life course of clients who are their patients. This interruption of a patient's contemporary and future life career means that hospitals must be properly organized so as to effect the chosen intervention. One implication is that the structural characteristics of hospitals can vary significantly *and* systematically, depending upon the hospital's orientation toward its patients.

Because hospitals can take contrasting interests in their patients, they induct more *or* less of the person into the organization and "keep" the client there for either a long or a short period of time. In the second chapter in Part III we indicate how this fact may influence the content of interpersonal relationships in different types of hospitals.

Finally, the last chapter in this final Part explores some implications of the client biography perspective for inter-hospital relationships, especially as they bear upon questions raised earlier about collaboration and cooperation between hospitals.

The Epilogue deals with some questions about the future of medical care organization, especially as it may be affected by the intervention of public sectors of medicine into the private sphere.

Like so many other books, the writing of this one has no easily discernible starting date. Both of us have had the interests reflected in it for quite a long time. As a result, we want to acknowledge our indebtedness to all who had a hand in molding our interests—teachers, colleagues, and friends—long before we actually sat down at the typewriters. At the same time, the ideas explored here—especially those in the latter half of the book—can be traced to earlier work done by others as well as ourselves.

More recently we have exploited our friends and co-workers at the University of Rhode Island and at Case Western Reserve University in examining some of the ideas set down here. It would be impossible to name all of the people with whom we had lengthy discussions. Some would probably choose to remain anonymous anyway.

Our students have been especially helpful. Like most good students they gave us some very hard times indeed. Rosengren taught courses in complex organizations in 1966, 1967, and 1968, and these were at times geared toward wringing out some of the ideas explored here. Lefton directed several dissertations which moved toward an extension and operational measurement of some of these thoughts and their application to organizations *other* than hospitals.

Mrs. Gloria Sterin and Miss Germaine Dennaker served amiably and well as research assistants, and their library and editing efforts were invaluable. Miss Elizabeth Pratt of Narragansett prepared the final manuscript and we thank her.

Eliot Freidson originally encouraged the idea, edited the manuscript at various stages, and kept us going when we fell into writers' slumps. It is not mere etiquette to say that the defects of the final product are due to our stubborn refusal to take his advice now and then. Whenever we took it, the result was improvement. We are truly indebted to him for his graceful style as a consulting editor and for his friendly counsel.

Acknowledgment is due also to the Division of Community Health Services, United States Public Health Service Grant CH-00289, which partially supported the work reflected in this publication.

Finally, our families have been helpful and forebearing: Our wives by sometimes taking exception and sometimes by refraining from doing so; the smaller members by being more quiet and immobile than children really should be.

WILLIAM R. ROSENGREN
MARK LEFTON

PART ONE

THE TWO chapters in this first Part introduce the dual themes traced throughout the book. The first theme is the very practical and pressing problem of how to maximize the availability of current health care resources and technologies. The second focuses more upon the issue of how the sociological perspective may be exploited, not only to yield satisfying explanations for the relationships between health organizations and patients, but also to keep abreast of increased health needs and rapidly burgeoning new experimentation in health care delivery.

Chapter 1 deals specifically with the scope and magnitude of health needs and problems in contemporary society and some of the dilemmas posed by the facts of increased health care expectations among the population, the objectively true increases in medical technology with which these expectations can be met, and the awakening awareness of the inadequacy of our present and dominant systems of health care delivery—the lone practitioner on the one hand, and the short-term general hospital serving bed patients on the other.

Chapter 2 surveys some of the recent efforts to counter this inadequacy by altering traditional and existing forms of health care organization. These have ranged from an intensive utilization of emergency room services, to home care services, health team approaches, comprehensive care, ambulatory care, and regionalization of all medical facilities in a geographical area.

Throughout all of this emerges a picture of a growing concern with bringing the organization of health care more in line with newer conceptions of what the patient is, or might be, as a partial "member" of the hospital system. This last issue raises, of course, a multitude of practical problems with which medical personnel did not have to contend before. It also raises an interesting sociological problem: How can we understand these new attitudes of the patient on the one hand and the hospital on the other?

1
Hospitals and Patients: An Overview of Issues

No longer merely infirmaries for the shelter of the sick poor, hospitals have become scientific institutions, key instruments in the provision of twentieth-century medical care. Since hospitals have become the definitive place in which modern medical care is given, they have the major responsibility for demonstrating new ways of patient care.

GEORGE A. SILVER, "Social Medicine at the Montefiore Hospital"

The critical roles played by large scale organizations in the contemporary scene prompts the writing of this book about hospitals and the persons who take an active part in them— patients included. In an indirect way, it is about other organizations which see as their *raison d'être* the provision of service to clients. We focus on hospitals and their patients for several reasons, including the fact that more and more people experience hospitalization during their lifetime. When they do they usually expect to be treated both effectively and decently. These joint expectations are related to the many different and newer modes of medical care recently developed. The results of these organizational responses to client demands are yet to be adequately assessed.

Going to the hospital is a deeply felt event in the life of a human being; it also reflects some important drifts in contemporary Western society. The expectation of efficient and thoughtful care appears to accompany increased urbanization and increased democratization of access to *all* principal social institutions. The extension of the concept of the long and good life seems to accompany affluence and modernization everywhere. It is not surprising, therefore, that medical organizations are increasingly impelled to devise new ways to satisfy human health needs. That these efforts are not instantly successful may be accounted for by the limits of medical and administrative science, and by the unanticipated contingencies which always characterize human institutions.

One remarkable paradox of contemporary society is that while modernization increasingly takes the character of a technological order, it is also marked by an ethic of humanism. Accordingly, the social establishments which mobilize the technological resources of a society seem always to be informed by an ideology which holds that while man's needs are probably best served in an efficient manner, they ought also to be attended in a kindly fashion. The paradoxes deriving from technological efficiency on the one hand, and the humanizing concerns of modernization on the other, are most discernible in formal organizations—hospitals especially. Thus, the study of hospitals is pertinent in that it serves to highlight the central dilemma of modern complex organizations—technological efficiency versus humane service.

The contradictory biases which are inherent in the social study of human institutions are apparent in Robert Redfield's claim that a notable drift in modernization is increased dominance of the moral over the technological order, that *relationships* between men as strategies for control are increasingly more salient than is mere *manipulation* of men by tools; while Thorstein Veblen, with equal vigor, heralded the coming dominance of the "engineer," and thereby prophesied the ascendance of science and technology over and above ideologically based social institutions. Both may be right in the context of medical organizations which must now address themselves to both historic imperatives.

Hospitals are of interest in that they embody in dramatic

form these two central institutional patterns and because they are directly in contact with those who receive services: clients.

A focus upon the client provides a vehicle by which to bridge conceptually the gaps between several hallowed theoretical traditions. Specifically, there is a long-standing preoccupation in the social sciences with the points of contact between the individual and social organization. The influences which each brings to the other have been characterized and phrased in a variety of ways. The sociological repertory has for a long time contained conceptions such as primary and secondary groups, formal and informal organization, *Gemeinschaft* and *Gesellschaft*, universalism and particularism, folk-urban, sacred and secular, and other dichotomies.

The similarities of these typologies derive from a felt-need to dramatize and to name alternative outcomes of the confrontation between the individual and the social system. Although they all contain this central element, the empirical referents include various levels of the social organization, ranging from whole societies to concrete interaction between individuals. It is precisely in the context of formal organizations that the confrontation between the person and the group can strategically be studied. First, because formal organizations are manageable empirical entities—less than society but more than family. Further, formal organizations manifest all of the major contemporary societal drifts: bureaucratization, depersonalization, professionalization, urbanization, etc., all of which have their imprint in organizations.

In summary then, an explicit focus on the client-patient, especially on the way he is defined by the organization, serves as a device to address three interrelated tasks: how to understand structural variation in organization; how to assess the impact that reacting clients have upon organizational dynamics; and how it happens that organizations extend themselves in various ways beyond their doors.

Until recently, prevalent ways of understanding complex

organizations—and of constructing them as well—have stemmed largely from a consideration of the techniques and values of industrial and administrative enterprises. This concern with exclusively "technologically" oriented institutions—as seen in their rational orientation toward their work, their insulation from external social forces, and their structurally precise ways of accomplishing tasks—appears to be confronting a changed emphasis. Organizations may now be more sensitive to societal expectations, geared to greater flexibility in the strategies of work organization, and attempting to implement the judgment that the multiple demands of clients may call for organizational criteria which no longer fit with an older conception of bureaucratic rationality. However successful has been the concern with organizations in their rational aspects—both analytically and heuristically—this approach has failed to encompass a fuller understanding of organizations manifesting a dual allegiance to both technological and humane criteria. In other words, organizations dealing with the social and personal dilemmas of individuated man may be less satisfactorily served by a conception of organizational design and analysis stemming from a consideration of purely technologically oriented institutions.

This book deals with the impact that clients have upon the operation of formal organizations. In it is set forth a framework for understanding client-serving organizations which may be useful not only for hospitals but for other kinds of complex organizations as well.

THE EXPANDING ROLE OF HOSPITALS

General Health Needs. That hospitals play an increasingly important role in the life of persons is patently true. It is instructive to record some of the ways in which hospitals, health needs, and medical services preoccupy not only the time but also the resources of contemporary society.

Of all expenditures for medical care—including doctors' fees, dental costs, and medications—hospitals claimed nearly 88 per cent during the six-month period ending December 1962.[1] The dollar dominance of formally organized ways of providing medical care is further supported by the fact that of all forms of medical expenses, it is the least sensitive to all those socio-demographic characteristics that normally *make a difference.* For example, while the per capita expenditure for dental care *decreases* markedly with social class position, expenditures for hospitalization remain very nearly the same regardless of class position. Further, while hospital care absorbs over 90 per cent of all medical expenses for those in the six-to-sixteen-year age group, the amount of money devoted to hospital costs decreases to only 85 per cent for those over sixty-five. This seems to be true in spite of the increased use of various medical insurance programs. The effect of Medicare is yet to be assessed in mediating the continued cost of hospital care through the life cycle, and as a strategy for "total" care of the aging.

Stated in yet another way, 1,000 persons with less than five years of formal education will probably visit a physician— usually in a hospital or clinic setting—about 400 times a year and will experience about 129 discharges from a hospital every year. People holding a college degree will probably visit a doctor—in a formal medical setting—about 540 times each year and be discharged from a hospital about 125 times annually. Apparently hospitals and illnesses do not discriminate by social class or age, in spite of all the efforts to ameliorate the health needs of the disadvantaged. The problem may be even further exacerbated by the fact that organized medical settings, clinics and hospitals, *do* seem to claim comparatively *more* of the illness time and medical care resources of Negroes than whites.

It is instructive to keep in mind the changing age shape of the American population and the increasing urbanization of the society in order to appreciate fully the ubiquitousness of hospitals, and to comprehend what the future might hold as far as the relationships between hospitals and patients are concerned. The young American is taken to a doctor about six times during his first year of life, and only two or three times at age ten. He consults a physician more frequently each year from that age until he reaches seventy. From then until he dies he is likely to see a doctor about seven times each year. Among all age groups, visits to doctors are somewhat higher in urban than in nonurban areas, and are even more frequent in highly urbanized regions of the country than in small communities.

This increased "democratization" and "urbanization" of medical care can be fully appreciated only by the degree of specialization repeatedly shown to have accompanied the urbanization-modernization process. More and more persons now receive medical care in formally organized places with the attendant routinization of task, universalism of criteria, and specialization of function to which the fact of complex organization has customarily led. Visits to clinics increased by about 50 per cent between 1958 and 1963; home visits declined by about the same magnitude. The effect of class and caste is to be noted here in that the "organized medical contact rate" for non-whites is about *three times* that of whites,[2] suggesting that the formally organized hospital as the main locus of modern medical care may be a mixed blessing for an increasingly vocal segment of the population.

Total Patient Care. Hospitals and other organizations have recently been exposed to the expectation that since they have gone far in perfecting their main technological repertory, they ought also to expand their services and therefore to incorporate more of the "total patient" than was once thought to have been feasible. Hence, client-serving organizations address themselves to the humanistic theme by offering

services on a broader base. The result of this for organizational efficiency and client satisfaction remains a moot point.

Chronic Care. The *long-term* involvement of medical institutions with their clients seems to be a joint function of the
changing demographic shape of the population and of the
felt capacity of medical technology to treat ill persons on a
long-term basis. It has been estimated that about 74 million
persons suffer from some form of chronic illness. Of this number, somewhat more than 18 million suffer from some form
of activity limitation traceable to their chronic condition.
Furthermore, about one and one-half million chronically suffering people are disabled from their usual work routines.
Nearly 10 per cent of those suffering from heart conditions
or arthritic problems cannot work. Finally, about 6 per cent
of the 74 million (not a meager number when viewed in ab-
solute terms) experience a major activity limitation of some
kind. This simply means that the men cannot work, and the
women cannot care for their homes or their families as they
have usually done.[3]

No one seems yet to know just how many older persons
with a chronic illness are institutionalized. Certainly a large
number are—there were well over half a million in institutional settings in 1963. Of this number, slightly more than one
half were resident in places under proprietary sponsorship;
others were in nonprofit and government institutions. That
the hospital as a unique form of institutional care is becoming
more and more to be the last home of the aged-chronically
ill is surely noted in the fact that while the number of nursing
care beds increased by less than 3 per cent in the twelve-
month period 1962-63, the number of hospital beds for the
chronically ill increased by nearly 10 per cent in the same
period—more markedly so in the proprietary group. Propor-
tionately, there were fewer hospital beds added among non-

profit institutions. But in governmental institutions, usually the largest of all, the increase was quite significant.

Whatever is the precision of the figures, it seems likely that the chronically ill person in his later years is more and more likely to find himself in the care either of a small proprietary institution or in a large governmentally sponsored organization. In either case, Leonard Mayo's contention is important: The small private institution seems subject to operational control by its sponsoring group however capricious that control may be, while the large governmental organization is bound by the bureaucratic constraints on operation inherent in its far-flung administrative commitments. The effects of both forms of control on technical-humanistic orientations toward their aged-ill clients can be manifold.

A Place to Die.   There is of course that final human episode of dying. Though it may be true that the hospital is no longer regarded only as a place to die, it is still the case that in 1956 about 63 per cent of all hospital discharges in the Middle Atlantic part of the country were made as a consequence of the patient's dying there.[4,5] In sum, nearly 75 per cent of all dying persons experience this rite in formally organized settings which have their own strategies for dealing with the social psychological contingencies of death. This figure can be interpreted in at least two ways. First, it indicates the efficiency of our medical system in that terminally ill persons tend to be routed to that organization best equipped to handle their fate effectively. It may, on the other hand, indicate that hospitals are faced with the need to deal in the best ways they can devise with a human experience that has no efficient or easy technological answer.

A recent national mortality study revealed that about 88 per cent of all deaths occurred in a hospital setting.[6] This ranged from a high of 95 per cent for those in the birth to forty-four-year age groups, to a low of 83 per cent in the sixty-five and above group. Moreover, females tend to die in hospitals rather more frequently than do males. In spite of the fact that a large number of those who die in hospitals do so on the first day of admission, a not insignificant proportion are patients in a hospital for a quite long period of time before their lives are lost.

In Sum. If one were to set forth in broad outline the importance of hospitals in the lives of people, one way of so doing would be to consider a composite of the organized health service experiences of the typical American: Life begins in a hospital and he sees a doctor rather frequently as a child. Visits to the doctor taper off during young adulthood; then they increase markedly as he grows older. All of this is likely to be more pronounced if he lives in a city. The proportion of his financial resources spent for hospital care will remain quite constant regardless of his age, sex, or condition in society. Even if he is poor, he is likely to experience just about as many hospitalizations as is his more comfortably endowed fellow citizen. Thus the hospital system is, in the main, blinded to capacity to pay. A mean condition is likely to result in less frequent and less expensive care of his teeth, purchases for medicines, and all other forms of health care. Though he may carry some form of medical insurance, the fact of being insured is—perhaps surprisingly—likely to result in more rather than less frequent hospitalization and higher rather than lower expenditure for hospital care. This may well demonstrate that not only are medical organizations geared to provide more and more expensive care, but also, that an increasingly large segment of the population want and expect more medical care. And they seem to take whatever steps are available to secure it, regardless of the cost.

If an American lives to old age, thus taking part in a well-documented demographic drift of the present day, he will see his doctor less and less frequently in the home and more often in a formally contrived organization such as a hospital or a clinic. If he is fortunate enough to live to be old, he runs the risk of surviving only with a chronic illness of one sort or another and chances are then about one out of ten that he will be disabled from his work and home responsibilities. The probability is great that such a contingency will result in even more care and supervision through a formally organized medical establishment. Finally, whether he lives a long or a short life, in all probability his dying will be guided and organized in the nexus of the hospital world.

The facts are repeated here to illustrate that hospitals are of increased importance in the lives of those whom they serve.

CHANGING ENVIRONMENTS
AND THE SHAPE OF INFLUENCE

Social trends are affecting the traditional relations of hospital and patient in other significant ways. Hospitals have come to occupy a rather different place than they once did in our social-psychological life space. Oswald Hall has remarked that an aura of magic and mystery no longer envelops the hospital, and patients increasingly confront the hospital on its own rational and sometimes disenchanted terms.[7] Not only is medical care now viewed as a citizen's right to which patients may lay claims, but doctors and nurses are increasingly regarded as persons who have their own private interests at stake, and these must somehow be accommodated to the demands of the healing arts. While hospitals consume more of available societal resources, patients now seem to present themselves for treatment in a less compliant posture than they might once have done.[8] In short, patients must now be "contended with" if the hospital is to accomplish its goals.

There seems little doubt that hospitals are increasingly important to those who work in them. Given the argument that work is indeed the central life interest of professionals and that medical care is increasingly professionalized and specialized it is logical that the consuming world of work is increasingly located in large-scale organizations. As Warren Bennis has argued, the proliferation of work careers in complex organizations seems to have enhanced the worker's involvement and investment in his work rather than diminished it.[9] This is probably as true for hospital employees as for others.

The local communities in which hospitals are located, and the sometimes antagonistic power cliques of which communities are composed, have a stake in what hospitals do. For hospitals, and all client-serving organizations, are at once the servicers and the servants of the local community. If there is an increased democratization of the receipt of medical care, an important corollary is increased pluralism in the control and guidance of such organizations.

The importance of hospitals is marked by the growing "nationalization" of health problems and health institutions. It may be true that "We move toward the welfare state but we do it with ill grace, carping and complaining all the way."[10] Still, the percentage of the gross national product devoted to health matters rose from 5 per cent to nearly 8 per cent in 1960; federal government expenditures for health purposes rose from 13.7 billion dollars in 1955 to nearly 33 billion dollars in 1965.[11] Indeed, the increased participation of the federal government in the human affairs of local communities, in all spheres of service, is a fact so obvious as to require no further comment. Large-scale federal programs such as Medicare, urban renewal, and the many specific welfare programs subsumed under the Office of Economic Opportunity seem often to have confronted local communities with potentialities with which divisive organizational complexes in the fields of health and welfare have been unable to cope. Hence the externally imposed demands for interorganizational collaboration among local community health services are but a further complicating ingredient in the relationships between medical organizations and their clients. For as service organizations such as hospitals have arisen in response to the particular needs and demands of special segments of the local population, so too the total organizational system in metropolitan communities has developed a remarkable capacity for the delivery of service against this backdrop of interorganizational divisiveness and even conflict.

The dilemma lies, of course, in the fact that newer federally initiated programs in the fields of health demand a degree of collaboration and integration of which few communities seem as yet to be capable.

Hospitals are of interest because they touch the careers of people, both employees and patients, in many ways and often for a very long period of time. Some of these impacts highlight significant changes in the social order, especially as they reflect accommodations between technical efficiency and humanism as organizational criteria. Also, they are a critical focus through which one may observe shifting relationships between formal organizations and the local community, on the one hand, and between organizations, communities, and the national polity on the other.

It has been said that a distinctive hallmark of the hospital context is the unavoidable confrontation between personal need and professional zeal.[12] It may be useful to point out the many important consequences of the existence of a professional and administrative line of authority in hospitals, but the pattern of conflict may well take the shape of a triangle if patients are included as active participants in the life of the hospital. Although under some circumstances administrative authority may lead to pressures toward a hierarchical order of authority, and the professional line toward colleagial relationships and the maintenance of individuated though affectively neutral relationships of the organization toward its clients, the patients are more likely to oppose both administratively inspired bureaucratization and professionally-based cool detachment.

This does not compel the conclusion that professionals in hospitals always constitute a united front *vis-à-vis* the administrative perspective, nor are they always in agreement about how patients ought to be handled. In fact, the more technologically elaborate hospitals become (surely to be more the case in the future than in the past), the greater will be the number of different medical specialists employed. Differentiation of function seems always to result in differentiation in social origins, social interaction, in commitments, and in orientations. Participation by patients in the life of the hospitals may well join in one important way with increased technological sophistication and professional complexity—namely, allocative decisions (judgments as to what resources in what amounts shall be devoted to what purposes) may increasingly be made by administrators. This is necessitated perhaps by the negotiative processes obtaining between multiple professionals, with the demands by patients to control their organizational careers as a further exacerbating factor. As a corollary— perhaps partially because multiple-professionals must be engaged in ordering their relations with one another—the emotional tone of hospitals may be defined in the future by the expectations of the patients *and* outcome of negotiative processes between the professionals.[13]

Thus hospitals are *prima facie* ubiquitous in the contemporary scene. They are of massive economic importance not only in the national economy but also in the private budgets of individuals. They are an important locus of technological and ideological innovation, precipitating the former and reacting to the latter. They are of profound interest as places which manifest social change perhaps even before such changes make themselves known in other organizational spheres. They concern themselves with some of the fundamental values of modern society—the maintenance of life, support for the incapacitated, and guidance for the dying. With the possible exception of aerospace laboratories, they are the most professionalized of modern formal organizations and mark the significance and joint confrontation of compassionate concern for clients and of the ethic of scientific manipulation of materials. They epitomize the community institution in their allowance for a clear demarcation of the boundaries, and their permeation, between the host community and its satellite organization. Yet in spite of the historical association between hospitals and their community settings, they are the one client-serving institution caught up at most junctures with the drift toward nationalization of both the technics and values of humane care. And most germane to the thesis to be developed in this book: Exceeded perhaps only by the college or university, hospitals are organizations in which the collaboration—or at least the passive acquiescence—of the client is most mandatory in the delivery of the service. As a consequence hospitals may be viewed as an organizational archetype in which clients play a most dramatic and critical role not only in intraorganizational structure and interpersonal dynamics but also in the outcome of current demands to effectuate meaningful interorganizational collaboration. Hospitals bear some of the prophetic imprints of the times. Yet they are, separately, sufficiently unique in their purposes, their forms of organization, and in their relationships to their clients to provide the curious social scientist with a rich array of organizational types.

PLAN OF THE BOOK

Following this general overview of the changing role of the hospital on the current scene, Chapter 2 traces some of the adaptive innovations by which particular hospitals have attempted to deal with explicit aspects of the problems they confront. To do so it becomes necessary, first, to consider the point of view of the hospital as one kind of unit in the medical care spectrum, and second, to recognize that in making adaptations the hospital is tending increasingly to act in conjunction with other hospitals or with medical colleges and to reflect both particular community trends and broader social developments.

Part II considers the sociological theory and research pertaining to hospitals up to the present time, and some of the diverse frameworks within which sociologists have attempted to organize their studies and interpretations. The position is taken that one logical approach to the literature is to categorize it according to the empirical referents which are the primary foci of the separate studies. Three major referents are isolated and assigned respectively to Chapters 3, 4, and 5. The first is concerned primarily with the internal structure of the hospital as a complex organization; the second focuses on the patient in the hospital and his interaction with other patients, staff, and structure; the third is concerned with both community morphology (i.e., the effect of the community or environment on hospital structure) and the interorganizational patterns existent and emergent.

Part III introduces a new frame of reference, suggested as a potentially heuristic device in unifying the multiple approaches to hospitals in particular and service organizations in general. The organizing empirical referents for the chapters in this section parallel those utilized in Part II—i.e., Chapter 5 focuses on the internal organizational dimensions and features of hospitals; Chapter 6 has the patient as its major referent; and Chapter 7 reconsiders interorganizational problems and prospects in the light of the same conceptual framework.

2

New Forms and Trends
in Medical Care

Out of chaos has come a time of crisis. . . . In the ideographs
of the Chinese language, two characters are used to write the
single word "crisis"—one is the character for "danger" and
the other is the character for "opportunity."

NATIONAL COMMISSION ON COMMUNITY HEALTH SERVICE,
Health is a Community Affair

THE COMPREHENSIVE CARE CONCEPT

Conflicting forces in the American scene converge upon
the hospital with jarring intensity. Urban depersonalization, technological specialization, and increasing costs conflict with more humanistic themes which seek personalization,
total and quality care for all. There is acute awareness of
these incompatible pressures on the traditional medical care
system especially in hospitals. Doctors, professional associations, and study commissions debate the relative urgency of
these several problems and the merits of proposed solutions.
But hospitals must deal on a day-to-day basis with the realities of too few beds, funds, staff, and unclear objectives. They
must contend, too, with a patient population growing more
impatient and angry about the discrepancy between mounting
health expectations and the realities of available health care.

This chapter seeks to define these problems as hospitals
now confront them. The forms of comprehensive health care

innovations now appearing will be examined and related to the problems which they address. Questions of over-all co-ordination and control will ultimately encompass these arrangements into a total planning pattern. Hence it is necessary to learn what has been done—meeting with both success and failure—before mass and imposed innovation begins in earnest.

Comprehensive Care and the Hospital in Action. The hospital today is caught on the horns of more than one dilemma. On the one hand, it is a practically oriented institution where serious medical ills are treated and to which individuals with a wide range of problems are routed. At the same time, the hospital has been forced to attack socio-medical problems which are not in clear accord with its traditional orientation. Whether such attempts stem from growing pressures upon its resources or from a sense of obligation to actualize its role as an instrumentation for all medically relevant matters, it appears that the hospital *will* remain the core facility in the medical care system.[1] As new problems are incorporated in the medical sphere, and as new responsibilities are delineated, it is the hospital which must serve as the spearhead of change and resolve.

This institution, representing the traditional view of medicine as a technically proficient and crisis reducing endeavor, must now promulgate newer medical ideas and practices only indirectly related to its primary orientation and objectives. The hospital is called upon to manage the chronically as well as the acutely ill. It is being called upon to prevent as well as to treat and cure; the hospital is increasingly relied upon to provide continuity of care and service, and to extend its reach beyond the ward and operating rooms into home and community. Perhaps most difficult of all, the hospital is to be the catalyst by which extra-hospital medical facilities are coordinated so as to deliver "total" medical care to those who require it.

In some quarters the notion of comprehensive care involves essentially changing conceptions of disease. Weinerman, for example, argues that the traditional model of disease requires severe modification in the face of social-environmental pressures and of several obvious but neglected changes in the patterns of disease per se.[2] He points out that illness in our society (1) is the predictable outcome of multiple environmental hazards (e.g., smog, speed, and the sheer weight of numbers); (2) is essentially nonpreventable (i.e., risk factors seldom act as single causative agents); (3) is often nonspecific ("the social diseases of our special environment permit no simple nosology and the number of demonstrable diagnoses varies with the patient's age"); and (4) produces a variety of manifestations that interfere in life functions over long periods of time (the chronic diseases are quickly replacing the acute, episodic illnesses as the key medical challenge).

A major conclusion is that medicine now requires a conception of illness which emphasizes "early" care, a "reaching out" of the medical-care system into the apparently healthy population or into segments of the population with known risk of disease. Newer models of disease must focus on its presymptomatic stages, its manifest symptoms, and its long-term prevention and care. What is generally called comprehensive care assumes great significance in the light of a pragmatic dilemma confronting medicine today—namely, the discrepancy between the *potential* capacity to produce effective health services and the *actual availability* or delivery of such services to those who need them. To further complicate matters, the notion of what constitutes proper delivery includes not only availability of facilities and personnel rendering services but also the manner and method by which medical procedures are organized and managed. More to the point is the increasing concern with who and what the patient is as a person.

In other words, availability and "style" are closely integrated features of what medical care is to be. Together these provide guidelines for evaluating existing delivery systems.

It could be argued with some justification that comprehensive care is perhaps more appropriately characterized as a perspective or even a philosophy than as a detailed program for action. But it is obvious that the concept has jarred medicine partially lose from its status quo mentality and has been instrumental in prompting some serious soul searching. While notions of comprehensive care are themselves reactions to profound societal changes which have exerted great pressures on the medical profession to re-evaluate traditional concepts, procedures, and relationships—these notions are both responses to and precipitants of new thinking and concomitant experimentation.

Although this discussion of comprehensive care is sketchy, it should be apparent that the concept casts a wide net in terms of its potential impact on virtually all aspects of medical training, administration, financing, and practice. The very diffuseness of the concept serves to leave no stone unturned. Whether this proves to be its virtue or its downfall, the fact remains that the medical profession *is* indicating great concern about a wide variety of issues that simply have not been scrutinized with zeal for several decades.

Although the special focus of this book is on a single (albeit major) facet of the medical-care system—the hospital—the scope implied by newer medical concerns and conceptions compels a consideration of that institution in terms of a frame of reference that transcends a parochial interest in the hospital per se and demands a conceptual model that more clearly relates the hospital to conditions and circumstances beyond its doors.

The Emergency Room as an Indicator of Stress. In a practical sense, the hospital emergency room functions as a visible barometer of the changing medical scene. It dramatizes the decline of past procedures and orientations and heightens the realization that the old was not nearly as effective as many are willing to believe. Also, the emergency room has underscored the need for medicine to recognize that existing methods and policies are antiquated and that sharply new procedures are demanded if medicine is to provide service in accordance with its principles and objectives.

According to an American Hospital Association report there has been a national increase of 175 per cent in emergency room visits between 1954 and 1964.[3] Among the factors cited as causing this increase, two would appear to be of major significance: the mobility of populations with large concentrations of low-income groups in metropolitan areas, and the unavailability of personal physicians in those communities, due to the specialization drain.

A study sponsored by the Yale University Medical School provides some supporting evidence. The study followed some 2,000 consecutive visits over a two-week period in an effort to assess factors affecting emergency room utilization. It was concluded that as the hospital becomes more of a community center, the emergency room plays an increasingly important role. It has become a basic source of medical care for economically depressed individuals and a back-up resource for the self-supporting when private care is unavailable for whatever reason. The findings also showed a pronounced class differential in the study population—a clearly defined tendency for higher proportional usage by lower socioeconomic groups. Of great importance was the finding that there was an irreducible degree of use of the emergency room for nonurgent medical care. That finding is not unique to the Yale study. Its repeated disclosure has served not only to highlight the inefficiency of such utilization but also to show that many thousands of persons suffering from nonurgent but nonetheless serious medical problems obviously have nowhere else to turn even though they may be acquainted with such alternatives as do exist.[4]

It is precisely at this point that demonstrable facts and the recent interest in comprehensive care are clearly complementary, and exert a dual influence on the hospital to reconsider its role in the medical system as well as to plan for pathways to resolutions of existing and future medical service problems. The hospital must more adequately screen persons and their illnesses to obtain more efficient utilization of the medical services it offers. The growing shortage of family physicians means that the hospital must provide its own preliminary diagnostic procedures. Where this first-line evaluation is to be done is problematic.

Hospitals, already overburdened and understaffed, are also essentially crisis-oriented institutions. These characteristics are ill-suited to many patients and to the systematic evaluation of all presenting problems, especially those more functional than organic, and those more suggestive of future trouble than indicative of immediate problems.

This is not to deny the accomplishments of outpatient departments. But the vast majority do suffer from the staffing problems already noted. Moreover, such facilities are usually adjunctive rather than integral functional aspects of the hospital, i.e., they are generally ancillary. Traditionally, this has been viewed as desirable, but the fact that the outpatient department staff and the hospital staff are one and the same often turns an adjunct facility into a peripheral and less important one—short-changed in organization, power, and priority. In short, the "real" business of the hospital is in the treatment of severe medical problems, and utilizing staff for a completely different medical service results in unhappiness for both staff and patients.[5] Medical personnel, especially students and residents, are motivated to deal with serious disease manifestations, and the general minority of such problems in outpatient populations often results in a style of care which, while perhaps medically sound, is negatively perceived by the recipient. The cold efficiency of the outpatient department often exacerbates an already medically alien mentality on the part of many patients.

It becomes apparent that an orientation to comprehensive care allows few problems to remain isolated. The great problems encountered by hospital emergency rooms are serious matters not only in themselves, they are integrally tied to a host of other important issues. There is concern with adequately meeting the needs of those who require emergency room treatment as well as those in need of medical help and attention who belong somewhere *other* than in that finely tuned facility.

Comprehensive care negates the idea that the hospital serves only those patients who physically present themselves for service. A chief feature of comprehensive care is the effort of the medical-care system to reach out into the apparently healthy population or into those segments of the population at known risk of disease. In short, a major future concern will be with the presymptomatic stages of disease. Many of the thousands of persons who turn to the hospital emergency room and outpatient departments represent but a small sample of the much larger populations that the cloak of comprehensive care is designed to include. With regard to the dilemma of hospital emergency rooms, these arguments suggest that such facilities will not and cannot be used appropriately until there is a complete system of medical care otherwise available that is "personal, continuous, and comprehensive." From the perspective of the larger medical system, the issue is just how this kind of care is to be provided, without sacrificing the technological gains of the past half-century. From the point of view of sociology, the issue is how to mobilize available conceptualizations in order to understand these newer forms of care and the unanticipated consequences to which they may lead. We move now to a consideration of a few of the more notable efforts to devise medical systems of this over-arching kind.

RECENT EXPERIMENTS

The Division of Social Medicine at Montefiore Hospital in New York and the Aging Center of the Sinai Hospital of Baltimore are two examples of recent efforts to enlarge the comprehensive elements in individual hospital service; that is, to incorporate as viable objectives a wider range of functional goals.[6] In both instances the hospital is the locus, the planner, and the purveyor of the core elements of comprehensive care. In the case of Sinai there is explicit reference to coordination and stimulation of outside resources to provide expanded service by demonstrating a need for them. It is important to note that for both hospitals the concern with innovation is relevant to two types of patients who many say present the greatest challenge for medicine in the years ahead. These two patient groups are often singled out as those most in need of total or comprehensive medical care—the chronically ill in the case of Montefiore, and the aged patients in the case of Sinai of Baltimore.

Social Medicine. The Division of Social Medicine at Montefiore Hospital represents a new willingness to adapt a broader role, facilitated by the nature of the patients involved.[7] Mainly addressing problems of a chronic type, Montefiore usually admits patients at a point where acute disease has been stabilized and rehabilitation processes are paramount. Both of these demand more patient and family participation in treatment, because the outcome is highly dependent upon patient attitude, family readiness, and general community support.

The pressures of long-term illness account for the Social Service Department and the Home Care Program. In its own right, the Home Care Program stimulated the idea that the hospital ought to provide medical service "both inside and outside the hospital walls." This in turn led to the family Health Maintenance Demonstration, an experimental program which tested many ideas of comprehensive care. By virtue of funding through H.I.P., the Division did not dissipate regular hospital resources, but could still implement an ongoing delivery system for the purpose of assessing the value of novel ideas in medical care. Hence, the importance of research in the delivery process was recognized and an evaluation of the program was viewed as an integral facet of the system.

A major finding was that permissive access to the hospital did not lead to an abuse of medical services. In fact, group patients utilized specialists less frequently than did the control group. Members tended to prefer the composite general practitioner, available through the team approach. While the physical health of member families showed greater improvement than that of the controls, their emotional health showed little improvement. Many families seeking care only for organic health problems exhibited the same symptoms found in those who sought psychiatric help but resisted referral for this purpose. They did, however, accept team counseling, and the then-Director, Dr. George Silver, suggested that this has important implications for professional manpower distribution.[8]

A final and important finding was the patient's greater acceptance of the public health nurse in place of the physician, and the warm reception afforded the social worker on the team. The public image of the social worker as a specialist was found to interfere with a capacity to use the service easily or early. A related discovery by Freidson was that a "lay referral" system had far-reaching implications for the ways and speed with which a family utilized the new medical service. That is, social and cultural factors in the community milieux of the patients did, in many instances, inhibit the speedy appearance of patients at the hospital.[9]

The Aging Center. This Center represents another attempt to bolster treatment facilities to meet more adequately the goals of comprehensive care. The patients selected for special consideration were persons whose medical needs were so intertwined with social and emotional problems that they could not be met effectively within the usual context of a general hospital—aged, indigent, and chronically ill persons. The Aging Center of the Sinai Hospital of Baltimore was formed in 1961 to investigate in depth the special problems and needs involved in the aging process and to define appropriate methods of dealing with them. The first step was to set up an Information and Referral system located in the hospital but available to the entire community. Under the supervision of a trained social worker, the service was designed to provide patients and hospital alike with a ready reference to community-wide services offered to the aged.

The medical arm of the Aging Center, the Medical Services Department, is located in the hospital's Out-Patient Department. Patients are assigned to one physician and seen in his "office." This "personal physician" does the initial work-up and is responsible for continuing care thereafter. Consultations are made available as required through the regular specialty clinics. An essential feature of the program is that the personal physician attends the patient when admitted to the hospital or even to the home care service. To support the work of the personal physician and the aims of the Center, special attention is given to Group Counseling and Recreational Therapy —these are developed early in the program with the recognition that the aged suffer greatly from loneliness and depression.

Perhaps the most innovative aspect of the Aging Center, and which so critically reflects the conception of comprehensive care, is the Home Care Service. This service admits patients in much the same way as does the typical inpatient department but defines eligibility as:

Non-ambulatory patients needing both medical and para-
medical service but [not] the more expensive facilities of
the acute hospital. . . . [Admission is from] Sinai Hospital's
service beds but also from the comprehensive ambulatory
clinic, from the Emergency Room on occasion, [and] by
application, from private physicians and other hospitals.[10]

As in the case of Montefiore, evaluation is a core element
of the new program. A careful assessment of the Aging Center
after three years of operation revealed the following:

1. The costs of the program are high but a positive element
must be noted as a result; namely, staff has become more economy oriented, an attitude reflected in selectivity in the use of
laboratory services. "As physicians in the program have become more conversant with the problems of aging, the costs
have come down."[11]

2. Familiarity with aging problems has also helped young
internists on the staff to become more comfortable with their
role in chronic and terminal care. House staff is involved to
the degree that medical residents rotate through the program
and are introduced to the underlying philosophy of long-term
and home care. That is, by virtue of the Center being an
integral feature of the hospital, training and education have
been expanded to include professional interest in areas beyond traditional boundaries.

3. Attending staff increasingly have tended to utilize the
Information and Referral and Home Care Services. Not only
is such usage of benefit to patients but hospital beds are
utilized more effectively and economically. In fact, hospital
capacity has been expanded without increasing the actual
number of available beds.

4. A critical consequence has been the delineation of special
needs which has triggered recognition of certain inadequate
features of the hospital's care system. For example, the Center
has stimulated expansion of the Hearing Clinic and has

prompted the cooperation of outside agencies to bolster that particular service.

5. While the evidence is still somewhat fragmentary, it seems that neither hospital admissions nor home visits have been required as much as would be expected ordinarily for this type of patient population. This has been attributed to the emphasis by the Center staff on meeting needs *as they arise* and preventing major problems from developing. It is also the case that the program has undoubtedly increased a sense of security and confidence on the part of patients to manage more effectively on their own. The drop in referrals to nursing homes and chronic hospitals provides substantive support for that judgment.

Home Care Services. It seems reasonable to argue that a key development of both programs just described is Home Care Service—medical service delivered to the patient in his or her home. Furthermore, in both instances great attention was paid to establishing the service as an inherent feature of ongoing hospital operations. Home Care has become in both institutions more than an adjunct service ancillary to the main business of the hospital. The importance of such service to patients cannot be underestimated, while at the same time it offers a series of superb opportunities for medical education in accord with recently espoused objectives of comprehensive care. According to Rogatz and Crocetti,[12] Home Care offers an incremental education factor not duplicated in most other services. Specifically, staff and students from all hospital disciplines have the opportunity to observe and contend with problems of illness as they affect patients in their natural settings and to assess interactive processes as they affect and influence the progress of specific illnesses.

A second significant educational advantage stemming from Home Care Service is that interdisciplinary cooperation is learned much more easily. While staff is drawn from several disciplines their allegiance is to a common service directed at the same patient. The management and medical problems stem from the patient rather than from diverse specialties and there appears to be less interference from barriers of differential orientation and a greater tendency to draw from each the assistance needed to achieve an over-all team aim. It is argued that such experience enhances an appreciation of what can be attained by the mutual pooling of skills. This leads to a clearer understanding of both the limitations and the capacities of each discipline and increases appreciation of external cooperation among disciplines and services as an indispensable part of the practice of medicine.

While Home Care does serve to reduce the need for both acute and chronic hospital beds, the economy involved is somewhat misleading because much of the time allotted to patients under home care would not be allotted under conditions of traditional inpatient service in most hospitals. It is critical, however, to assess carefully the economy involved in home care service primarily because of the ready expedience measure it can offer as a "dumping ground" for unwanted patients rather than as a selective alternative mode of appropriate care. Maximum benefit is obtainable by treating the program as an expansion of hospital facilities, personnel, and teaching programs.

It is evident that home care medical service for the types of patients of Montefiore and at Sinai is both desirable for the patients and functional for the staff. But it must be emphasized that the desirability of such service is critically dependent on the nature of its relationship to the hospital proper and its basic orientation and operations. More specifically, the problem appears to be tied to making home care services as medically significant in the eyes of professional and para-medical personnel as are the traditional and heretofore more glamorous and status providing aspects of intra-hospital work. In view of the growing importance in numbers and in medical complexity of an increasingly older population in our society, it is of the utmost importance for future research to probe the implications of such services for the patients, for the staff, and for the potential impact they may have on the structure and functioning of hospitals.

The Health Complex as Core Facility. While definitive research on newer forms of medical and hospital care remains to be done, an examination of some views on the shape of things to come provides insight into possible implications of efforts to promote more effective medical care for greater numbers. For example, *Medical News* quotes Dr. William Hubbard, Dean of the University of Michigan Medical School:

> The hospital has outlived its usefulness in its present form and must be replaced by the "health complex." As the main locus of patient care, hospital costs have risen beyond tolerance. In addition, size, numbers, and varieties of personnel tend to dull the fine point for identifying responsibility for the patient . . . and promotes routines established out of necessity for efficiency . . . [to] deal with patients in very similar fashions even though their needs may be very different.[13]

The health complex, Hubbard suggests, would concentrate diagnostic and treatment resources in ambulatory services, self-care units, extended care and convalescent units, all oriented toward preventive and continuing care to a total patient group. It would appear that the proposal is for medical service to be arranged in units according to criteria informed by the requirements of patients rather than in accord with traditional hospital disciplines and services. Such emphasis on the patient and his needs would give rise to a series of decentralized, self-contained, and administred units and would apparently function in a way quite different from current hospital wards attempting to provide similar services.

Dr. Hubbard is pointing to a need for specialization in an

important sense but not in the customary medical sense. His concern with specialization derives from the needs of patients and the structural arrangement for effective delivery of care. This would be based on a network of semi-autonomous functional units rather than on the tight, formally arranged ward or service units now found in our hospitals. In order for the medical system to meet the multifarious needs of patients new institutional arrangements must be developed. These arrangements should be developed not in the mold of the most successful of all medical establishments—the hospital—but rather in terms of the needs of patients.

The Health Complex idea, therefore, is an approach to medical care quite different from those of individual hospitals trying to innovate and expand their resources and facilities. In terms of potential impact, it is indeed a marked advance over what appears to be the modal medical reaction to newer pressures and demands, such as the relatively contained efforts on the part of hospitals like Montefiore and Sinai, which retain control and autonomy while expanding in terms of similar but internal functional differentiations. More specifically, it appears that each hospital, rather than expanding or adapting its resources to meet the demands of all such problem medical groups as the chronically ill, the aged, various population segments at special risk, home care service, etc., would instead remain functionally specific. That is, the hospital would continue to serve the acute and episodic disease and illness manifestations and would leave the service and care of other types of medical problems to other organizations. In the ideal, such facilities would be autonomous, structurally and functionally, staffed by medical and para-medical personnel with status equal to those serving directly in the hospital, but viewed as integral and cooperative agents in a larger medical care system.

The Medical Center today approximates the concept of a health complex but generally lacks the finely discriminated functional distinctions called for in this ideal. Usually the medical center consists of a collection of hospitals characterized by special service orientations (obstetrics, pediatrics, etc.), and is generally bound to a university medical school for educational and consultative needs. It is often the case that such networks are health complexes in name only. However, as they extend into the wider community by virtue of affiliations with community hospitals and other service agencies for either service or research purposes, the notions of the health center become more viable as practical aims. In other words, a group of affiliated hospitals and agencies begins to realize the aims of a health complex as it collectively develops and integrates amublatory care services, preventative measures, joint education programs, multiphasic diagnostic screening measures, and home care service. As the system begins to show concrete attempts to coordinate operationally the multiple services and agencies as relevant features of medical care, the actualization of a core health complex may be in the making.

Like the concept of comprehensive care, the idea of a health complex suffers from a lack of clearly defined organizational details. However, there are a number of concrete developments designed to pursue actively what appear to be the manifest aims and objectives of this new and potentially radical style of medical care delivery. The intrinsic features of such programs vary considerably—especially in the kinds and scope of patient problems to be served. But once again such empirical attempts may foster delineation of procedures, techniques, and structures about which the concepts alone are still obscure.

The Yale–New Haven Medical Center—Family Health Maintenance. In 1965 the Yale University Medical School launched an experimental program designed to develop and study new methods in the provision and teaching of family health maintenance.[14] The emphasis was very much as in the Montefiore Demonstration on achievement of comprehensive care through treating whole families as "patient." In this case the organizational framework and staffing reflects a more complex external differentiation. The scope of the program was extensive, but its patient population small. It was to promote family health maintenance through broad orientations to prevention, treatment, rehabilitation, and assumption of responsibility for coordinating patient use of related community agencies as required. The service facility is considered to be a self-contained, organizationally separate unit of the University Medical Center. While physically located on hospital premises, it is properly viewed as located in the heart of the neighborhood being served.

The educational function of the program is realized by medical students, under preceptors, leading the "health team . . . in place of a solo physician." Each team retains its own patient group but occasionally team members may belong to more than one team. Continuity of care is stressed with specialist consultation available. Several external agencies provide personnel for service at the center—e.g., public health nursing, welfare representatives, social workers. All complex medical problems uncovered can be referred to resources of the parent hospital complex.

For the sake of achieving maximum coordination in practice, the planning of the entire program involved a committee of community health agencies as well as a committee from the medical center. Financial support was obtained from the Office of Economic Opportunity and the local Community Action Program. Central to the operational aims of the center was the principle that policy commitment and program support was pledged by the cooperating parties.

Although the program has not been operational for long, the patients and families involved are offered an impressive array of medical care and treatment measures. The patients served are, to this date, few. Hence, the concentration of services is not altogether surprising. An important question is whether such a program can be translated directly into large-scale service facilities involving large numbers of individuals. Notwithstanding the lack of such knowledge, the concept of neighborhood health services associated with a medical school represents a positive venture in provision of a style of medical care more in keeping with recent views and orientations than the older traditions.

St. Paul Medical Center—Coordination of Community Resources. Whereas the Yale–New Haven Medical Center is deliberately small-scale in its operational aims if not in conceptualization, the next report examines a program in which the operational scope is the diametric opposite.[15] The St. Paul Medical Center is a nonprofit organization, formed in 1960 by five hospitals combining their outpatient departments and some aspects of ward and teaching services as a nucleus for their respective graduate medical programs and a special service facility for indigent patients. In the interest of comprehensive care for these persons, community resources of a wide variety were considered as vitally linked to the program. An intensive program was undertaken to coordinate center activities with those of all other agencies from which and to which patients were referred. This measure involved a concentrated effort at orienting staff to total patient needs, policies, programs, and problems of the many health and welfare agencies used as auxiliary resources. Every effort was made to interest the agencies in participating—literature was developed and inter-agency conferences on mutual problems were encouraged.

A report on the program after six years of operation comments that the coordination problems among the several participating units "have been met vigorously but not with complete success . . . the forces of specialization and apathy remain strong."[16] It is clear that the effort to foster an orientation on the part of medical personnel toward "the skillful appraisal of the total patient" . . . and to gain "the undiluted cooperation of community health and welfare agencies" has met with limited success.

In St. Paul there are 120 separate health and welfare agencies, governmental and voluntary, federated and independent, religious and charitable. Some are subject to national headquarters, others are local to autonomous. The vast problems in coordinating on a purely voluntary basis that number and variety of agencies, some of which saw little need to cooperate, are obvious if not completely understood. Despite discouraging reports, the St. Paul attempt remains committed to the proposition that the kinds of needs being met by the external agencies are absolutely critical for comprehensive care. The difficulties in operationalizing that goal are severe and provide indications of the tasks ahead.

These brief comments of ongoing efforts to meet current medical challenges, while obviously failing to provide the substantive materials for purposes of evaluation, do reveal several critical matters relevant to the place of the hospital within a total medical care delivery system.

First, there must be greater specification of what is said to constitute a "total medical care system." We have shown that the scope of medical systems, despite their expressed aim to provide comprehensive care, ranges quite widely. It was the neighborhood in the case of the Yale–New Haven Medical Center; it was the "total urban community" in the instance of the St. Paul Medical Center. It is apparent that the types of operational and administrative structures pertinent to each program varies greatly. In the former it is clear that the university hospital is primary in decision-making. It provides the core staff, the consulting services, and maintains control of the principle staff members because they are students in the university medical school. Those community agencies whose advice and help was needed were actually "co-opted" into the planning and operation of the project, and also, since the operation was small, referrals were handled on an individual, personal basis. The hospital in this case has little need to be intricately involved in a decision-making process which extends too far beyond its doors.

On the other hand, in St. Paul the medical center represents a different danger. Given the community orientation of the center and the fact that no less than five separate hospitals were instrumental in launching that program, it is apparent that the decision-making process is fraught with a host of difficulties not at issue in the Yale experiment. These are obvious conditions to be sure—the delineation of what such problems are in terms of their specificity, priority, and critical importance for the sake of success or failure, is another matter.

A second significant trend concerning the nature of a medical care system has to do with the attempts on the part of individual hospitals to expand their own services and to make their resources available to a wider range of medical problems. It would appear to be the case that the hospital-focused system is more restricted in scope than are those informed by medical or health centers which pointedly attempt to utilize external services and agencies. But the communities in which hospitals are located simply do not always have available external services. If they do, they may be but letter-head facilities without a viable work force or operational program. In short, the social setting in which a hospital is located greatly influences the innovations attempted and suggests clearly that they must be taken into account in any attempt at understanding plans, programs, and successes or failures.

Experiments in Regionalization. An early example of a regional amalgum is the Pratt–New England Medical Center (comprising in 1960 some 59 community hospitals, extending from Boston, Massachusetts to Maine and Connecticut).[17] The Medical Center was begun by the affiliation of two large hospitals with Tufts Medical College and Dental School. The first satellite hospital was at Rumford, Maine. The connection began with an informal series of lectures for Rumford doctors on new techniques and technologies given by a carefully selected Center doctor.* Maine patients with complicated problems were referred to the clinic. In turn, the clinic sent house-staff out on rotation to teach and aid in diagnostic problems. The crucial relation here is *between hospitals* rather than between hospital and patient. Indigenous local hospitals and physicians in smaller towns command a more general loyalty and confidence than is common in urban circumstances. The prestige of the New England Center would not impress the more rural resident as much as his urban counterpart, and would require the endorsement and referral of the primary service practitioner to a far greater degree.

The underlying objectives of the Center physicians were based on extension of urban advantages in quality medical care to rural patients. The problem was seen as one of aiding the isolated practitioner with limited facilities, to bring him "back into the main channels of medical progress." Tact and understanding were needed to unite the existing and complementary factors of a patient population with developed local services, known, trusted but limited, with the complete medical facility, the source of information, specialized competence and technological machinery, but alien and potentially threatening to local autonomy and pride.

While the principle of raising the quality of patient care guided the over-all process, the day-to-day steps toward implementation attended to the exigencies of local practice, local

---

* It is worth noting the stature of the man selected to do this introductory and actually exploratory job—he was later to be a Medical Director of the Center itself.

influence, and fear of usurpation. There seems to have been no haste, and the greatest flexibility of approach. The broad objectives were gradually and skillfully translated into the terms in which they were meaningful to those having the ultimate power of acceptance or rejection, and expanding cooperation was confined to and informed by the areas in which needs became recognized.

Approaches to Ambulatory Care. In Hunterdon County, New Jersey, another project was launched, also informed by the new ideas of design and operation.[18] Two notable innovations in the Hunterdon program were the Ambulatory Service and the association of general practitioners, working on a fee-for-service basis alongside board certified but salaried medical staff specialists. The Ambulatory Service was not based upon patient capacity to pay and did not require bed care in the hospital. The fee-for-service arrangement with the general practitioners provided patients with access to a reasonably low-cost and well-staffed hospital complex.

The Hunterdon program represents a successful mobilization of community effort and interest in providing quality medical services. It appears that the citizens of the County backed up their committee members by a grassroots fundraising campaign reflecting enthusiastic support of the "service" concept upon which the experiment was based. In fact, it was this service orientation which transformed the Ambulatory department of the hospital from a free substitute for private office practice and a source of captive "teaching materials" to an alternate mode of care for all, limited only by the nature of the service required. Hunterdon County stands as an example of the development of working associations between an innovative change in the medical system and the surrounding community organization.

Unfortunately, the Kalkaska County, Michigan, experience represents a failure in this regard. This was an attempt to bring quality and innovative forms of medical care to tiny communities in rural Northern Michigan. After a three-year period of operation, the study group for the project found little community appreciation of regionalization as a positive asset. On the contrary, community isolation and self-suffi-ciency was more preferred. McNerney states, "Regionaliza-tion had no prior roots [in the community] . . . without the prestige and financial backing of the Foundation . . . [region-alization] agreements could not have been conceived. . . ."[19]

One village had new beds, but it had neither public health nurses nor a home care program. Joint purchasing, tried by only one center, was dropped after six months even though it had resulted in a 15 per cent saving on supplies. Regional hospital administrators had come faithfully to local hospital board meetings and had offered sound advice; they were politely received and promptly forgotten. There is a long cata-log of good ideas that passed through the system without leaving a trace.

If there was lack of communication between the program sponsors and indigenous community leaders, so too was there an inadequate formulation of the administrative structure of the new system. McNerney's description of the Board meetings reveals an organization so small that none of the evils of bureaucracy are to be found; nor any of its rational efficiency either. The conduct of hospital affairs was completely in-formal, with ad hoc decision making and no planning ahead.

Perhaps the most important lesson to be learned from Kalkaska County was that only the role of the town hospitals was made clear and effective. The functions of other segments and sectors of the medical system were ill-defined, vague, and equivocating. In the absence of effective leadership and guidance, most of the constituent members of the regional plan merely took what they felt they needed from the system, while the main content lapsed by default.

Regionalization of medical services may be the next large-scale development. Hunterdon, in fact, was conceived as just such an experiment. A vital component in it is a close affiliation with the New York University–Bellevue Medical Center. It is autonomous in all locally contained aspects but has a "permeable boundary" which permits free exchange with the large urban complex for educational and research advantages.

One evident characteristic common to all regional plans is that they tend to grow from a central and highly specialized facility rather than to arise spontaneously from an amalgamation of scattered facilities. Further, there seems a need to "woo" smaller units into the larger organization by subtle inducements based on their own most acutely felt needs. Failing this, the inescapable impression is that hospital autonomy is too highly prized for any part of it to be willingly or easily relinquished.

THE NEW MEDICAL SYSTEMS AND THE PATIENT

These newer forms of medical organization—all arising as a response to the call for comprehensive medical care—alter not only the traditional relationships between separate health organizations but also the standard relationship between medicine and the patient. Each particular innovation—whether it be ambulatory care, home care, preventive medicine, or what have you—necessarily limits the *number and kinds* of interagency and medicine-client relationships which it can serve. Each innovative form may do little more than contribute to the existing segmented pattern that characterizes the American medical scene.

Regionalization by federal mandate, however, may presage a genuine systematization of medical care. There are more and more medical procedures so costly, so demanding of refined and scarce skills, and so infrequent in need, that it makes little sense to provide them in every community. They are more appropriately located in centers of concentrated technology, research, and other highly specialized services. But patients from a wide referral area must then have access to these facilities and the means to use them.

There is emerging a picture of the future involving a set of facilities moving from the extremely rare and complex system, to those requiring intermediate type hospitals less widely separated and specialized for the larger number of people who are likely to require them. The primary level of facility is likely to perform functions exactly opposite to those accomplished at the highest level of medical sophistication. Primary facilities are effective when they are quite small, neighborhood based and oriented, broad in scope of interest in patients but shallow in treatment depth. Here, the majority of cases do not require more specialized treatment services, but do require breadth of understanding, intimate knowledge by the practitioner of family and environment and of pertinent social and cultural variables. The emerging ideal for the primary level includes the fewest possible types of medical practitioners, who offer to a limited number of families virtually unlimited supervision and guidance in health affairs.

There is also a need for formal linkages with external agencies which supply the same patient population with *other* health and welfare services. It is at the point of relations with external agencies and agents that accommodation to local needs and local community settings is most critical and potentially disruptive of new medical systems.

Toward a Synthesis. These novel forms of reorganization clearly reflect the fact that the medical world is beset today with profound challenges. Major changes are in the making, both from the standpoint of the individual hospital and from the perspective of entire communities. A major point at issue is that those who analyze from a sociological perspective, and those whose efforts at medical reorganization are being analyzed, can no longer afford the intellectual luxury of denying the orientations or conceptual predilections of the other. Efforts to understand the contemporary health scene must not only look toward building a common base for projections as to what the future might bring but also set forth, in broad outline, the fundamental issues involved. Moreover, there must be a *rapprochement* between an analytic starting point and a concern with specific medical elements, issues, and problems.

Hence, the problem before us has to do with how to set forth the necessary conceptual devices which will serve to relate systematically the three foci alluded to earlier: (1) the problems of specific medical organizations, hospitals particularly, in an organizational-administrative sense; (2) the role of the patient for whom specific agencies and systems exist, and to whom medical care is delivered; and (3) problems of interorganizational linkages in the fields of health.

In large part, this book sets forth just such a conceptualization. It is a reaction to and modification of existing theoretical approaches to hospitals; at the same time it seeks to address the practical realities of today's medical scene. Many of the studies and reports of hospitals suffer not so much from defects in problem definition, methodology, or conclusion, but from an isolation and lack of integration with *other* studies. This situation is similar to the isolation and separateness characteristic of the medical system itself. In general, the existing literature on hospitals, and to a large degree what passes generally as medical sociology, is better characterized as the accumulation of discrete and segmental aspects of the field. What is called for is a conceptual point of departure which permits *both* systematic analytical comparisions between and among different kinds of hospitals *and* a sensitivity to and responsiveness to the practical medical issues of our day.

In the literature to be examined in the next three chapters there are widely scattered clues that crisscross analytic definitions of hospitals, patients, and communities. We will examine these as a summary statement of existing concepts that tell us a great deal of *separate* areas, but which are difficult to grasp at once.

We shall be concerned later with transposing these arguments and examples into propositions to determine the future nature and outcome of health services. Having before us, then, a summary account of the theoretical base of medical sociology—and relating this to our "transposed variables"—we shall attempt to show that they have a natural relation to one another when considered from a single and unifying conception. We think that what emerges is valid not only for hospitals but for other service organizations as well, since the common focus of all such agencies is the client to be served.

What *is* unique about hospitals as service organizations is that they have, in most cases, a highly developed technology by which work is done. Hence, they are different from other service agencies (schools, welfare agencies, etc.) exactly to the extent that a major focus is upon technological criteria and administrative efficiency. They drift toward production organizations. But while this is true to some extent, it is only partly true. If the "product" is a "patient," he, like any other client, is capable of resisting "transformation" and the entire "production" process. As a result, outcomes can never be fully predictable. The identity of clients as persons and the relationships thereby entailed should prove to be highly consequential across all perspectives of medical sociology and all types of service organizations as well.

PART TWO

THE THREE chapters in Part II examine some of the important studies of hospitals in terms of three frames of reference. Chapter 3 surveys a series of investigations which focus upon the internal structural features of hospitals as formal organizational units. A central and dominating aspect of this first set of studies is that all utilize, either implicitly or explicitly, the classic bureaucratic model of organization as the theoretical departure point. In contrast, Chapter 4 describes a number of studies distinctly different in character in that far greater attention is paid to the recipient of hospital services—the patient. Included here are several attempts in the tradition of social system analysis and symbolic interactionism as well as other theoretical frameworks which illuminate the dynamics of patient life and the vicissitudes of interpersonal relations in the formal context of health care and treatment delivery. Chapter 5 examines a group of studies—some discursive, others empirically concrete—which are organized around still another point of reference: the ways in which the single hospital is functionally related to other hospitals and health organizations in its environment. Interest in interorganizational phenomena emerges in distinctly different approaches, ranging from community morphology as the guiding perspective to examination of more formal ties between types of organizations.

To some extent the very logic of this classification begs one of the major questions with which this book is concerned—to specify the linkages by which multiple analytic levels are related. A major task in Part II is to discern commonalities across frames of reference as well as to sharpen distinct boundaries.

The designations of these three frames of reference is a relatively arbitrary choice from among many other alternative groupings. The one most frequently employed by investigators is merely the "type" of hospital examined. When one looks for the assumptions that may be implied in considering differences between types of hospitals, some peculiarities of focus and attention emerge. For instance, while nearly three-quarters of all hospitals in the United States are short-term community general hospitals, very few studies have been made of them. Similarly, the extensive literature on the internal structure of psychiatric hospitals deals mainly with extreme cases of two special types—custodial state hospitals and elite institutions. On the other hand, a disproportionately large number of highly specialized medical organizations have been studied—hospitals for children, for the treatment of exotic and terminal illnesses, and so forth.

In nearly every case, the generic form of service is emphasized as the primary determinant of hospital structure and operation. The types of services studied tend to be those which deviate in some marked fashion from more "ordinary" forms of institutional medicine. So we find much information about the constraining, restrictive, and goal-displacing tendencies of the state hospital, but little about the effects of state sponsorship as such.

The symbolic interactionists have paid more attention to staff-patient *conflict* than have others, but seldom have they distinguished between degrees and kinds of conflict in response to differences in hospital structure. In the morphological approach we find the general hospital studied in relation to its host community. Here the focus is primarily on the organizational and demographic links bridging hospital and community without reference to the internal structural properties of the involved institutions, or to the consequences these might have for interhospital relationships.

Delineation of the findings derived from these different perspectives will set the stage for an attempt to place them in a common context in Part III.

3

Hospitals as Bureaucracies

There are several important features of the bureaucratic approach to organizations in general, and hospitals in particular, contained in the assumption that organizations may be viewed as "microsocieties." From such a point of view, hospitals are assumed to be self-contained and to have definitive boundaries which clearly demarcate them from other social institutions. The microsociety approach to organizations is imbedded in the assumption that organizations are rational plans for the achievement of specific ends. Satisfactory criteria of efficiency constitute a further important element. These prime conditions are related in the following way: The presumption of definitive organizational boundaries is a prerequisite of organizational efficiency to the extent that the presence of impermeable boundaries enhances the rational pursuit of specific organizational ends. A third distinguishing feature of the microsociety approach lies in the fact that the classical Weberian conception of organizations does not contain the analytic tools required to incorporate either organizational operatives or organizational clientele. This is so because Weber's analysis of bureaucracy was geared principally to a concern with administration—*organization for work*—rather than to the actual *performance of work*. Hence a parody of such a study of hospitals would yield a description of a hospital unrelated to the larger social order in which it resides, which operates with reference to uniformly applied criteria of efficiency and rationality, which contains no doctors or nurses except as they are involved in the administration of work rules, and finally, a hospital which has no patients.

The historical fact that Max Weber was not really very interested in the relations between organizations and their clients in no way implies that his ideas have not informed many studies of hospitals and have not given rise to revised conceptions of organizations more directly concerned both with hospital operatives and patients.[1] Nonetheless, viewing Weber's work from the view of the sociology of knowledge, it is a fact that he wrote during an era when client-serving organizations were comparatively few in number and of minor societal importance. Insofar as Weber was concerned with formal organizations at all, his concern was with delineating the principal features of that type of organization which distinguished modern *administrative* authority from *other* forms of authority.

For several reasons, the ubiquitous bureaucratic model seems unsuited for the analysis of operational organizations in general and for relationships between organizations and their clients in particular. Yet the theme of organizations as bureaucratic microsocieties persists as a dominant one in the study of hospitals. In fact, a great diversity of hospitals have been examined consistent with the bureaucratic model. The prime concern has been with the operative-administrative personnel in organizations rather than with the clients served. This approach has yielded a large body of literature which compares and contrasts the internal structural properties of hospitals with expectations and hypotheses derived from the ideal type. Deviations from the ideal are generally explained by fixing, in an ad hoc fashion, upon factors and variables not contained in bureaucratic theory itself.[2]

The main features of Weber's classic conception of bureaucracy include a hierarchy of authority based upon official mandate rather than personal license; a clearly delineated sphere of authority; impersonal relationships between participants;

and a guaranteed career which presumably assures protection for the individual and exacts his loyalty to the organization.

Studies of hospitals which take such a conception as their point of departure tend to examine the ways and extent to which the hospital world conforms to just such a logically consistent pattern of organization, and then to explain why deviations from these norms do in fact occur. In spite of its heuristic utility, the bureaucratic point of view is inherently limiting in that consistent structure and a logically understandable cluster of organizational characteristics are commonly found only in some administrative-industrial enterprises.

Perhaps the single element which bears most directly upon the question of why hospitals seldom *exactly* resemble a bureaucracy is to be found in the oft-noted inconsistency in Weber's writings about bureaucracy. Weber tells us that authority in bureaucratic organizations resides in the hierarchy of offices *and* in demonstrated expertise.[3] Yet the larger and more complex an organization, the more likely is it that expertise will be held by persons outside the administrative line. In hospitals, for example, most administrators are not medical experts, and most medical experts are not administrators. One line of authority deals with organization for work, and another deals with the conduct of work. A recurring preoccupation of students of hospitals concerned with the "fit" of medical organizations with classic bureaucracy has been with the manner in which accommodations are made between the constraints of administrative authority and the demands of the free professional for autonomy.

The only way in which a large community can be medically served is by large-scale, complex organizations which, if not accurately characterized as bureaucracies in the "pure" Weberian sense, do certainly share with other existing bureaucracies many common internal requirements, external pressures, and modes of administrative and operative behavior. Communication, coordination, fiscal responsibility, continuity of policy and re-evaluation of policy across changing internal and external conditions—these features may have different priorities in different cases, but the fact of complexity in staffing and in function presents insistent claims which must be attended to in a hospital complex no less than in an automobile manufacturing enterprise or a large government bureau. While Weber may have excluded from consideration certain factors which are salient to service organizations (i.e., the client), this does not negate the features of his theory which explain and define the root requirements for the large-scale performance of tasks through specialized divisions of labor. Notwithstanding the inadequacy of bureaucratic theory for the distinctive aspects of service organization, it may be possible to locate systematic modifications of the theory which illuminate the implications of Weber's basic statements when appropriately applied to these distinctive features.

For instance, the purpose of hierarchy is communication, control, and the centralization of information for effective decision making and for the operationalizing of central decisions. The pertinent question is not whether the exact form of hierarchy seen in General Motors or American Telephone and Telegraph can work in a hospital, since it doesn't, but rather what other mechanisms have evolved and whether or not they do the job. There is also a question to be raised about the differential requirements for centralized decision making of different kinds of decisions, and where decentralization occurs, the degree and means of formal coordination.

With respect to "work rules" for example, we must consider that there are different kinds of "work rules" appropriate to administrators and their staffs, to physicians and their para-professional aides, and to the semi-autonomous professionals who perform interorganizational tasks for the hospital in the attempt to relate to external agencies. Nevertheless, there *are* explicit work rules in each case. When we turn to the "patient as the product," we have to account for the particular characteristics of this kind of "material." When we consider "tasks," we have to understand the nature of the total constellation of factors which impinge on and affect task-accomplishment. These are all different in the case of the hospital from that of the factory operation, but the common element is not to be overlooked: that efficiency and effectiveness are as important for each, although correctly defined in different terms and achieved by different means. No matter how different the task or the training of the operator, he still must interact with the administrative structure in such a way that the total operation has coherence, especially when a given single organization may number its employees in the hundreds and its turnover is high.

Finally, we must remember that hospital organization may vary from classic theory in some ways that are similar to those in which all modern bureaucracies do, first, because "ideal types" do not pretend to explicate all individual variations and, second, because the passage of time and progress has introduced factors whose impact must be accounted for and which help to distinguish what is generally true in the theoretical formulation and what is culturally and temporally specific. While it is essential to make the assertion that a hospital is more than *just* a bureaucracy, we may have to acknowledge that it necessarily is one form of bureaucracy in a highly elaborate technological form. Even if this is not taken into account, its effects cannot be wished away.

Some of the studies reviewed here focus on deviations from the classical model—how and whether the ways they deviate are specific to the hospital context or are more generally true of professional bureaucracies. Others point to the fact that the bureaucratic structure does in fact exist, and as such has dysfunctional consequences for effective task performance. In the latter case, the question is whether a large organization can survive without such dysfunctional bureaucratic features or whether the hospital must be split into smaller units amenable to other forms of organization which circumvent bureaucratic features. While there seems to be in the first case a preoccupation with "fit" between an existing model and actual hospitals, the second case attempts to do away with the model altogether. There may be a third alternative which adapts the model to suit new requirements.

For instance, the ideal of impersonalized relationships is a requirement for universalistic rather than particularistic criteria. If we tend to assign rewards by merit rather than by status, if we hold that all patients should receive good care regardless of capacity to pay at least in public or semi-public institutions, then this is *not* less the case because considerations of personality bear on the effectiveness of treatment. We do not rule out universalism per se because for specific and task-related reasons we deal with persons rather than with inanimate objects. Because authority cannot run in a straight line from an administrative head, there is little to be gained by denying that some sort of authority, of performance control, and of coordinated task governance exists as an essential aspect of all work.

BUREAUCRATIC STANDARDS AND PROFESSIONAL VALUES

Mary Goss studied and explicated the problem of dual lines of authority and suggested it need not necessarily result in conflict situations in hospitals.[4] By means of a single intensive case study she has drawn out characteristic features of the medical-control element and concludes that although it is different from customary administrative control patterns, it may be equally effective. She extracts the distinction between bureaucratic requirements in general, and the specific requirements of hospital-medical bureaucracy, formulating a tentative subspecies of the genus bureaucracy. It is becoming apparent from the related literature on this topic that the in-

tervening "species" is the professonally dependent bureaucracy which has increasingly to find or evolve new mechanisms
for reorganizing rigid administrative hierarchies to permit
specialized professionals the degree of autonomy they require
to apply the criteria of their respective disciplines without
disrupting the coherence of the organization as a whole.

Goss suggests that a distinctive form of bureaucratic authority is evidenced in the separate medical line within hospital control systems; this she designates as "advisory" authority. While doctors resist any extraprofessional interference in
medical matters, they do not form strictly collegial relations
among themselves as a "company of equals" any more than
they tend to conform to pure bureaucratic authority patterns. Rather they assume an intermediate position which
permits a considerable degree of control from the top, yet
permits the maximum autonomy compatible with competency.
This advisory authority rests upon desire for approval from
colleagues, which Goss finds to be a powerful determinant
affecting the behavior of doctors. Thus top staff men or attendants with demonstrated high competency legitimately
give "advice" to younger colleagues or internes, which is
accepted and in most cases followed. To follow advice is
not in itself mandatory. If an interne is convinced that some
immediate circumstance justifies alternative measures, he may
obey his own judgment, and a successful outcome will ensure
approval of this move. Even a mistake will not penalize him
unduly if his action was soundly based on the evidence and
on his best judgment. Here the impersonal rules are represented by technical knowledge; the negative sanctions are directed
against poor judgment and failure to know the rules—i.e.,
the basic theory and the practical medical evidence. Subordinate and superordinate alike share a common value base
which ensures a high degree of consistency and effectiveness
in this process.

Certain typically bureaucratic features are nevertheless

compatible with this authority structure which appears so flexible. There *is* a formal hierarchy of positions; impersonal or universalistic criteria are supposed to apply to hierarchical position and determine the "right to give unsolicited advice." Goss concedes some importance seems attached to formal ranking in the over-all organization, but finds no empirical evidence by which to decide the degree of its importance relative to that of demonstrated professional competence. She inclines to the opinion that among doctors in this country there seems to be more importance attached to reputed competence than to formal rank.

Discussing the work of Goss, Charles Perrow suggests that there is indeed evidence that the position of the doctor in a hospital bureaucracy is perhaps not as "deviant" as it might first appear. He points to the increasing professionalization of bureaucrats in all areas: "engineers, accountants, chemists. . . . The medical profession has a stronger grip upon its members and the specific hospital a weaker one. But the difference is one of degree. . . ."[5] He also points out tellingly that a good deal of professional medical knowledge deals with explicit rules for explicit circumstances, and that skill and judgment as well as "knowledge of rules" is required by all trained occupations. "Skill and judgment are the essence of 'advisory bureaucracy.'"[6]

Goss points out that in spite of apparently obviating the division of labor requirement, there may be considerable advantage in physicians assuming a part-time administrative function. Perrow takes this a step further and suggests that administration is more than just paper work; it is in fact *power*. He emphasizes that organizational goals, policy determinations, and implementation of change depend, in the long run, upon the administrative function, so that if the medical profession wishes to influence or determine the over-all direction of these forces, it will have to be more explicitly involved in administration.

These joint issues—participant control and the nature of the division of labor—have been extended by Rosengren in a study of psychiatric hospitals in order to examine their effects not only upon medical staff members but upon patients as well.[7] A distinction was made between control achieved through organizational structural means and through supervisory strategies. Those hospitals which emphasized "traditional" and technologically well-established modes of patient care such as electroshock, drug therapy, and other "physical" means tended to have rather formalized and specialized divisions of labor, hence obviating the need for close personal supervision of psychiatric-medical personnel. Control was accomplished through the division of labor itself, and the specific technological repertory which was employed. Other hospitals attempted to implement more "innovative" forms of therapy, which were less technically salient, such as group therapy, supportive psychotherapy, and other social means. These institutions contained more unspecialized diffuse and debureaucratized divisions of labor. Here structural controls were absent and broad and extensive personal supervision was used to maintain control over personnel. More important as far as the patients were concerned, however, is the fact that patients in hospitals containing minimal supervision of staff members were subject to pervasive and pointed control and supervision. Conversely, patients being treated in debureaucratized hospitals where staff members were exposed to broad supervision were subjected to *minimal* control. In Goffman's terms, the first were total institutions for the patients; the latter were total for the staff members. The evidence would seem to suggest that hospitals cannot escape the need to control their members in some fashion. Where bureaucratic strategy is absent, others are likely to arise. Perhaps more instructive, however, is the implication that the presence of staff members requires hospitals to elaborate one form of control; the presence of patients demands quite a different strategy.

The relation between administrative and medical authority is examined from another angle by William Glaser in a comparison of American hospitals with British and continental European models.[8] National-historic development of hospitals, the place of government in health services, and general economic and cultural differences are all seen as determinants of the greater emphasis upon administration in American hospitals than in their European counterparts. In analyzing this, he appears to define two quite different kinds of hospital units. In America, the hospital is characteristically autonomous, in regard to both finance and policy. It is complex and in a constant state of internal flux—new drugs are used, new techniques and technologies succeed each other rapidly, doctors are part time and mobile between several hospitals. In contrast, the European type is a relatively simple and slow-paced unit, deriving its simplicity by being administered externally as a public or denominational subsidiary and from being internally decentralized under powerful service chiefs who handle almost all matters pertaining to their own departments. Public hospitals are quite separate from small private hospitals which are usually run by doctors for their own paying patients.

Perrow, commenting on Glaser, thinks these distinctions are in part a function of different stages of cultural and economic development, and will gradually diminish.[9] He sees the bureaucratization of the European hospital as imminent, due to advances in technology, an irresistible force which impels toward size and bureaucratization. The greatest contrast to our system that he finds in the European system is the difference made between doctors who do most of their work in the hospitals and those without access to any hospital. Most American doctors do have access to some hospital for their private patients. Glaser sees this as a unique mode by which interprofessional quality control is exerted, since in the hospital the doctor's work is highly visible to his colleagues, and withdrawal of hospital privileges is an extreme form of sanction. But even this difference, in Perrow's opinion, is on the way out. He notes that increasingly there is a trend toward permanent, full-time staffing of hospitals in this country, at least for high-status positions, and more and more patients are being seen in the hospital setting.

While Glaser seems to suggest that the bureaucratization of hospitals is an optional development, it is the case in the United States because of pecularities of historical development and national characteristics (e.g., Americans have a natural tendency to "administer" everything in terms of industrial models). Perrow seems to be suggesting something quite different. In his view it would appear that it is the very nature of advanced technology and of the related economic power of patient groups which lead to certain features of size and complexity in hospitals that force the bureaucratic pattern. As the European economy and patient catch up with their affluent American counterparts, the same inevitable path may well be traversed.

Perrow attacked the problem of hospital bureaucratization by tracing the changes which occurred in Valley Hospital as it contended with its growth pattern over a period of many years.[10] The special problems attending the hospital during its early years resulted in domination by its patron groups. This initially gave the institution the tone of a community "mission," more responsive to the ethic of conviction than to the norms of rationality. Later, the medical staff achieved primary control, and in this era authority resided in the professional staff. With increased technological advances, control moved to the administrative branch with its subsequent bureaucratization. The determinants of this final stage appeared to be the many diverse internal and external groups and professions requiring coordination. In addition, medical specialization fragments the professionals, also calling for administrative control. Perhaps more important, with advanced technology, problems of obtaining and allocating resources become more and more an organizational problem. In each stage, different relations toward *client* groups predominate and the *client* group persists as a salient force effecting shifts in the hospital's internal organization.

Freidson and Rhea have concluded from their observations that relations between physicians in an American clinic setting tend toward those of a "company of equals," rather than what might be inferred from the formal structure of the organization.[11] Hence, problems of professional control are worked out in an informal and negotiated fashion mainly by "talking to one another." It has been observed, however, that while the "company of equals" pattern informs relations between physicians in most British hospitals, both it and bureaucratic prescriptions are modulated by an informal "hierarchy of age and experience" and professional maturity.[12] The difference may be a subtle but important one. In both instances, the full bureaucratization of the hospital is minimized by forces present in one country and not the other. In the American case, the salience of the professional norms may be greater than in Great Britain. But in Britain the impact of more traditional systems of rank and prestige may be present to a greater extent than in the United States.

An even more dramatic illustration of a hospital different from that prescribed by the bureaucratic model is found in the *Tsukisoi* in Japanese mental hospitals.[13] Caudill tells us that the incoming patient brings with him a female valet who tends to his personal needs during his period of hospitalization. The *Tsukisoi* is responsible only to the inmate and not at all to the official authorities of the institution. Such a pattern could hardly be tolerated in an American hospital, and probably reflects a very important contrast in the cultural definitions of mental illness in the two countries, as well as in the appropriate relationship between hospitals and their patients.

A case which looks *within* the hospital system itself in accounting for structural deviations from the bureaucratic model is found in Rose Coser's comparison of a general medical and surgical ward.[14] In relating the structures for work to the tasks of each type of service, it was found that the medical ward conformed more closely to the bureaucratic model with a clearly demonstrated hierarchy of authority from the residents to the internes. Autonomy in decision making at the nursing level was minimal. Specific "orders" and "commands" stemmed from routinized and standardized channels. On the surgical side, however, the authority system was considerably more flattened; the chief surgeon exercised autocratic and independent decision making. In spite of this, the line nurses on the surgical ward were expected to exercise more autonomy and inventiveness in their work than were medical nurses.

One way to account for these differences, both of which deviate from an ideal conception of bureaucratic authority, is to argue that medical wards often deal with illnesses that are difficult to diagnose and prolonged in time. In addition, the efficiency of chosen treatments must continually be assessed. Hence a feedback system characteristic of bureaucracy is an essential feature of the medical ward. Not only must orders be carefully channeled, and specific medical acts rigidly conducted and recorded, but observations as to results must be communicated in a reliable fashion to those who originally ordered them. On the surgical ward, the work target is more specifically defined, events occur rapidly, and outcomes are more immediately conclusive—even irreversible should they prove deleterious to the patient. Consequently, there is a shorter feedback line. Activities on the surgical ward are conducted in the pathos of urgency and crisis, and this often requires nurses to make independent judgments and take unilateral action.

Seeman and Evans also studied medical and surgical wards in examining how stratification among ward personnel influenced the performance of internes.[15] They found that less adequate medical performances were characteristic of the more highly and rigidly stratified wards. They also found a generally higher degree of stratification on surgical as against medical wards, but also significant differences of degree within each type.

The theoretical conceptions used in interpreting these findings were the ideas of "generalization" and "rigidification"—both of which resulted from high stratification. Generalization stems from the observation that high stratification among hospital personnel encourages staff members to generalize their attitudes toward the patient in accord with those held at the lowest level of the medical hierarchy. Conversely, low stratification allows for the diffusion of power and prestige more evenly throughout medical ranks. This, in turn, is thought to increase the likelihood that the patient will be included in the making of decisions affecting his treatment and disposition.

Rigidification refers to the tendency for stratification beyond optimum levels to become "an accretion, something adhered to not for its functional value but for its own sake,"[16] which leads to difficulties in communication and to the use of structures for "status ends."

In spite of these findings, the authors point out that while the differences were consistent, they were not as great as might have been expected. Two important explanations are offered: that the system itself has many "sources" of variance of which stratification is but one, and there is no adequate theory of stratification in relation to formal organizations which can be drawn upon in assessing these findings.

Considering the last two studies together, it becomes clear

that they have given rise to what might appear to be conflicting conclusions. Coser suggests that medical wards are closely akin to the bureaucratic model; Seeman and Evans show that surgical wards are generally more stratified than medical wards, hence more bureaucratized in this respect. In point of fact, an alternative explanation may lead to the conclusion that the actual differences are not that great.

There is, in fact, a finely tuned bureaucratic hierarchy, adjusted on each ward to the particular tasks involved. Within the context of both wards is the same rank order—head physician, resident, assistant resident, interne, and nurse. The distinction between these ranks may be blurred in situations where consensus and consultation are crucial, while rank distinctions are observed in high relief wherever specificity of function and procedure is the rule. The interne on a surgical ward is in the early learning stage. He is at the bottom of the performing ladder and observes most procedures, assisting only in a limited capacity. The nurse has far greater experience in the observation and routine care of the patient, and hence may appear to have disproportionate power as compared with the interne. The main medical tasks are performed by the chief resident or the assistant assigned to the operation, while the nurse sees to pre- and postsurgical care.

On medical wards, the interne is more often already in possession of knowledge which entitles him to make more decisions than his surgical counterpart, to participate in decision making with higher-ranking physicians, and to exceed the decision making power of the nurse. He is there being trained explicitly to *make* decisions, and is given limited authority to do so under advisory supervision.

Stemming from such an interpretation, it would be possible to make similar distinctions within other types of hospital wards depending upon the degree of specialization and the precise technology involved. For instance, it may well be that on an intensive care cardiac unit—even if entirely nonsurgical—an organizational stratification might be found which is more like the general surgical model than the medical model.

Blau's comment on the question of deviation from the ideal bureaucracy is pertinent:

> It includes not only definitions of concepts but also generalizations about the relationships between them, specifically the hypothesis that the diverse bureaucratic characteristics increase administrative efficiency. Whether strictly hierarchical authority, for example, in fact furthers efficiency is a question of empirical fact and not one of definition.[17]

BUREAUCRACY AND THE THERAPEUTIC MILIEU

Of special importance in specifying bureaucratic functions in hospitals, and especially their limitations as instrumentalities, is the research conducted in mental hospitals. The work of Stanton and Schwartz is highly instructive. In pointing to the deleterious consequences for patients stemming from conflict among the professional staff, these authors make the case that bureaucracy is dysfunctional for the attainment of mental hospital goals.[18] Their thesis is that certain bureaucratic features such as a hierarchy of authority and differential prestige in a clinical milieu create stresses and tensions which inhibit optimum therapeutic impact upon patients. In explaining this, it is first argued that mental patients are qualitatively different from the physically ill, and that psychiatric treatment itself requires more flexibility than does care administered to persons with strictly somatic diseases. In a word, a hallmark of the therapeutic milieu approach to mental patients is the emphasis upon particularism or individuation of treatment, as opposed to more universalistic and routinized procedures employed in nonpsychiatric settings.

Second, individuation demands a work context which fosters rather than impedes these goals. It could be argued that the traditional medical structures of hierarchy, status distinctions, clearly delineated lines of communication, etc., not only preclude particularistic patient care but also perpetuate dissatisfaction and unhappiness among ancillary and paramedical personnel, and that these also are inimical to the goals of therapy.

The logic of these arguments is: Milieu therapy involves a consideration of each patient's unique difficulties and needs, and requires a commitment to the patient as a person. The proponents of milieu therapy argue for status equalization, democratic decision making, and the promotion of an anti-bureaucratic organizational ethic.

Third, psychiatric patients are thought to be extremely sensitive to nuances in their environment. They are regarded as acutely aware (perhaps even subconsciously) of organizationally generated staff conflict and dissatisfactions, communication breakdowns, and the like. Very often, difficulties are traced to bureaucratic rigidities; hence they become targets for change.

An attempt to measure empirically the sensitivity of mental patients to these conditions and to appraise the effects of personnel tensions on treatment performances was made by Karras, Upjohn, and Lefton.[19] A situation was studied in which an attempted policy change in the hospital had resulted in a highly charged atmosphere. The findings were judged to be somewhat inconclusive because subjective self-reports were used and the number of patients involved was small. However, the authors tentatively suggested that they might in fact *not* be adversely affected by ward tension, either directly in the recovery process or indirectly by poor staff performance.

Notwithstanding the question of doubtful validity, the therapeutic community concept has had a profound impact in the ideology of mental hospitals, and even noticeable impact on the operation of many psychiatric hospitals. It has also had great strategic value for students of complex organizations in that it has permitted an examination of a hitherto inaccessible organizational phenomenon—the confrontation of competing organizational orientations in the context of the *same* institution. Specifically, the psychiatric hospital offers an especially useful locus for the study of the dynamics of bureaucracy because it exhibits a dual value system. The psychiatric hospital (like tuberculosis hospitals and others) contains a more or less rigid bureaucratic structure in the classic sense; the therapeutic community orientation attempts to subordinate traditional medical structures to the requirements of a warm, flexible, and conflict-free organizational environment. In such a context, status and power gradations would be minimal and decision making would be consensual rather than unilateral.

Lefton, Dinitz, and Pasamanick investigated the consequences of this duality for staff perceptions regarding their influence in decision making. The findings reflect the influence of both organizational orientations and raise a number of questions concerning the assumptions upon which therapeutic community policies are based.[20] For example, an effort to promote the therapeutic milieu in the face of an ongoing bureaucratized institution may give rise to a pseudo-democratic atmosphere in the clinical situation.

Observations of staff conferences revealed that nearly all decisions were made by the psychiatrists despite the conception of a therapeutic community in which all members of the clinical team participate in decision making. There were, however, interesting differences between wards in staff reaction to this situation. In wards oriented toward organic treatment, the staff on lower levels neither expected nor wanted to participate in decision making. But in wards with a strong psychotherapeutic orientation lower-echelon staff members did expect and want to exercise influence on decisions. As a result, staff members in lower positions in the psychotherapeutically oriented wards found themselves frustrated and less satisfied with the amount of influence they could exert than were those in organically oriented wards. It appears that the expectations engendered by a democratic ideology make low-influence positions even more unsatisfactory than they are in the *absence* of a pseudo-democratic climate. The commitment to a therapeutic community orientation leads personnel to believe that they will be able to exercise greater initiative and responsibility than they are in fact allowed to do. We do not suggest that bureaucratic features cannot be modified or changed. The point is that it takes a great deal more effort than many realize.

This brief review cannot recount all of the numerous studies of hospitals which take the bureaucratic model as their point of departure. Those cited, however, represent the major emphases of this research tradition. The fact that most hospitals resemble bureaucracies only partially may be explained by: (1) the impact of compelling cultural forces in the environment; (2) dual lines of authority (expert and administrative) require some modified form of bureaucratic authority; (3) nonroutine medical tasks seem to be accompanied by a less hierarchical form of authority than is customary in bureaucratic organizations; (4) a prime requisite of all organizations—participant control—can be accomplished by means other than a bureaucratized division of labor; (5) the special problems faced by hospitals in the delivery of service to the patients during the early years of their growth call for a distribution of authority inconsistent with the bureaucratic model; and (6) some of the ways in which hospitals deviate from the bureaucratic model may be the same ways in which all new organizations differ from older ones, and especially ways in which "professionalized" bureaucracies differ from others.

It has been pointed out that there is a degree of functional bureaucratization that does exist in all hospitals, and it may be less important to debate the semantic justification for the use of the term bureaucracy than to inquire into the degree to which existing bureaucratic structures serve the ends they are supposed to serve (rather than extraneous but ubiquitous external objectives) and what specific structures serve which specific ends.

For instance, both the community general hospital and the custodial psychiatric hospital have been said to be bureaucratic in nature. The first, however, seems to result in comparatively efficient care of patients, while the latter is more often regarded as treating patients with neither efficiency nor decency. However objectively true this may be, bureaucratic theory *does* allow for both contingencies. This may relate to the manner in which the administrative system accommodates to the professional ethic in the general hospital, while the operational line is more often co-opted by the administrative ethic in the latter. Such patterns suggest that although the objectively observed structures in general and psychiatric hospitals might be similar, a more important question has to do with how the participants actually conduct their work. This, in turn, would seem to lead logically to a consideration of two closely related factors: how clients are defined by the organization, and the way certain technologies are selected by which clients may be manipulated.

Frequently, however, the lack of "fit" between observed hospital reality and the classic bureaucratic model is explained by factors judged to be external to the hospital itself. This leads either to the social system or the community morphology approach, both of which tolerate deviation from bureaucratic theory. In general, clients of hospitals have no place in the bureaucratic perspective except insofar as they are regarded as "objects" to be worked upon rather than as "persons" with whom to contend.

4

The Hospital and Its Patients

A shift from a concern with the hospital as a classic bureaucracy to an interest in patients involves more than a simple
substitution of empirical referents. Involved, for example,
is a consideration of patients as "persons," and how patients
are affected by and themselves affect hospitals. As a result,
a special interest in patients requires a different set of conceptual tools from that which informs the bureaucratic perspective.

THE SOCIAL SYSTEM APPROACH

A case in point are those studies which stem from the
social system approach. Whereas the bureaucratic model assumes organizational autonomy, rationality, goal specificity,
and lack of boundary permeation, the social system perspective
rests upon the assumption that organizations have only analytic boundaries, not real ones, and that organizational autonomy is always problematic. Perhaps the distinguishing central
feature of the social system approach is the emphasis upon
system maintenance as *the* persisting organizational problem,
influencing the nature of goals which must be continually
renegotiated, and the manner by which inconsistent goals are
accommodated. From this vantage point, the hospital deals
with problems of maintaining workable institutional external
linkages and a workable balance among a variety of system
needs within arbitrarily conceived organizational boundaries.

Unlike the bureaucratic pursuit of a specific and *single* goal, the social system point of view focuses upon the variety of needs which organizations, hospitals included, must somehow satisfy if they are to survive.

Hospitals must strike a balance between the mobilization of available resources and organizational structures for the pursuit of instrumental goals (treating patients, maintaining employee commitment), expressive goals (supporting and maintaining the hospital's place in the cultural context of the larger society), and meeting the latent demands which both patients and employees bring to the hospital. In addition, hospitals must somehow maintain a balance between themselves as "special" institutions in society and as established representatives of the values and aims of the society at large.

Of specific relevance to patients is the notion that hospitals must accommodate between contrasting organizational demands and the orientations which individual participants bring to the hospital. While hospitals may maintain adequate primacy of instrumental functions, the patients may seek mainly emotional support and psychic gratifications.

The question of just how such conflicts arise is often attacked in an ad hoc fashion. Differences in socioeconomic and cultural characteristics between patients and staff is a commonly selected explanation. On a more abstract level, however, such conflicts may be regarded as emerging from a meeting of instrumental, expressive, and integrative needs—these needs resting upon a limited resource base. Hence, an "economy" arises out of which one of the three central modes of activity emerges as dominant. For example, system maintenance priorities may detract from the instrumental needs of the hospital. Under such conditions, goal displacement may occur. Furthermore, the pre-eminence of expressive needs, as against medically important issues, may lead to tactics by which the individual participants of organizations protect the integrity of their own personality needs at the cost of the avowed goals of the organization.

Some of the main features of hospitals, seen as social systems, have to do with the attempt on the part of their participants—patients as well as staff—to resist the depersonalization which attends organizational life. System maintenance, in particular, tends to exacerbate patient psychic stresses and strains in that hospitals when compelled to maintain their own security in the face of a sometimes hostile environment, often turn their work to issues only marginally related to the primary purpose of providing efficient and kindly care to the cure of the ill. Although patients *are* a part of hospitals, they have ranked rather low on the scale of analytic priority. They are affected by but seldom themselves affect the structural characteristics of hospitals.

Socializing the Patient. If the single most distinguishing feature of the social system approach is its emphasis upon the multiple goals hospitals must attain and the numerous functions they must perform, this complexity is further confounded by the variety of patient perspectives and expectations with which the hospital must contend. The nature of the systematic approach is stated clearly and simply by Coser: "The patient in the hospital . . . must accept the competence of doctors and nurses, must also adjust to social demands, some of which are not related to his 'getting better,' but to the maintenance of the social system."[1]

An important point throughout Coser's study of Mount Hermon Hospital is that the institution must somehow induct the patient into those roles and attitudes which will permit the hospital to address itself to its principal goal: the application of medical technology. These needs have latent consequences for staff behavior as well, as for example the exchange of macabre humor between staff members in moments of crisis. Hence, life in the ward may be described as in unstable equilibrium, a fact traceable to the need to socialize the patient as well as to treat him.[2]

The confrontation between the patient's primary, or expressive, orientation and the hospital's instrumental perspective is no better illustrated than by Coser's record of a medical interview.

> DOCTOR: When do you have pain?
>
> PATIENT: It's all here (pointing to stomach, chest, up to throat).
>
> DOCTOR: How long after you eat does the pain start?
>
> PATIENT: When I eat, like just now (points to supper plate). I eat a little piece of toast, a little butter with it, not much butter. Sometimes I take an egg, I don't eat much . . .
>
> DOCTOR interrupting: Can you remember being sick when you were a child?
>
> PATIENT: My mother had eight children (leans out of bed and takes her wallet out of dresser and shows her own childhood pictures). I had nine children myself (takes out another picture showing a man in uniform). That's my baby.
>
> DOCTOR WALKS OUT: I'll be back a little later.
>
> COSER: This patient's behavior would be appropriate for an interview with a psychiatrist, since the patient's expressive action conveys information that the psychiatrist seeks, but in the medical interview the physician's goal (a concise medical history) can only be hampered by the patient's expressive behavior.[3]

The processes of integrating these dual orientations—emotional support and technical intervention in organic illness—are also functionally related to the kind of therapy given: whether a mature physician or a "boyish" interne was in charge, the degree of responsibility imputed to the patient, and the extent to which the patient himself was expected to take part in making decisions about his fate.

Compliancy Theory. While not concerned exclusively with hospitals, Etzioni's theory of compliancy is a relevant theoretical statement.[4] Consistent with the social system perspective, compliancy theory stems from the proposition that the staff member's adherence to organizational rules, roles, and goals can seldom be taken for granted. Rather, it must be insured in ways that are consistent with the organizational structures involved. Hospitals, like other organizations, seem able to offer their members three kinds of inducements: symbolic, utilitarian, or coercive rewards. The first is identitive in nature and seeks to secure the worker's commitment by emphasizing the mission character of the work. This may also be buttressed by insignia of rank and prestige, ideological symbolization, and other secondary gains such as opportunities to associate with those of high rank and prestige. The second, utilitarian control, is primarily consumption oriented and involves wealth which can be expended for purposes not necessarily germane to the establishment from which it stems. The third, coercion, is the use or threat of force and is mainly deprivatory in nature.

Hospitals can be expected differentially to reward participants in these ways, and therefore to elicit contrasting kinds of worker compliance. Specifically, moral engagement is the bargain struck with those who receive symbolic rewards, calculative or instrumental involvement is the price to be paid for receiving utilitarian rewards, while alienation of members —whether staff or patients—is the fate of organizations using coercive strategies.

Etzioni contends that general hospitals are "tentatively" classified as symbolically controlling lower-level employees such as nurses, although there is little information concerning the ways in which patients are controlled.[5] The place of patients in the reward system of psychiatric hospitals is readily discerned: those in custody oriented hospitals suffer pain of coercion, while employees enjoy mainly utilitarian rewards. Patients in therapeutically oriented psychiatric hospitals appear to be the objects of symbolic manipulation, while nurses and other lower-echelon personnel are subject to more coercive manipulation. Referring to the work of Maxwell Jones and others on therapeutic milieux, Etzioni writes, "normative means of control are applied: informal talk, the personalities of the analyst or other personnel, and social pressures of the hospital 'community' including those of other patients."[6]

Not only are rewards differentially distributed among hospital members (thus telling much about the hospital's structure) but the activation of reward strategies is contingent upon the member's posture *vis-à-vis* patients. Those who must perform expressive functions (some nurses for example) are likely to seek symbolic rewards for themselves and to resort to symbolic means in order to control patients. Those who perform integrative functions (the hospital administrator as an example) are more likely to receive utilitarian rewards and also to use them in assuring the compliance of their subordinates.

If a hospital, general or otherwise, is organized in a hierarchy, those in the high positions are likely to receive both symbolic and utilitarian rewards, and to address themselves to patients in such a dual posture. Those in the middle ranks are likely to receive mainly symbolic rewards and to manipulate patients in similar terms. Furthermore, those in the lower ranks are subject mainly to utilitarian rewards (improved health, in the case of the general hospital patient) with the threat of deprivation (e.g., death) as a safeguard against lack of compliancy. Hospitals lacking hierarchical authority (some psychiatric hospitals for example) are likely to attempt compliancy through symbolic manipulation of both patients and staff.

The Hospital as Symbolic Worlds in Conflict. Some of the basic concepts of symbolic interaction theory—contact, interaction, and communication—may be drawn upon to point out the conditions under which patients and staff, though placed in the same context, actually construct symbolic worlds with contrasting values, meanings, and ways of accommodating to the constraints of organizational life. A distinguishing feature of this point of view is that organizations somehow are unnatural constructs which are counter to man's natural propensity to devise his relationships with others in an emergent fashion, without the unassailable limitations on conduct imposed by organizational life.

Thus, hospitals may be thought to be composed of two distinct social orders. There are those who regard the organizational property as their own and others who are there more or less against their will. Forced as they are into a direct interface in the contrived setting of the hospital, the relations between these two little social orders may be characterized by accommodation at best and open conflict at worst.

Because persons everywhere have a stake in the social worlds in which they live, the conduct of patients is likely to mitigate against their acceptance of curative efforts of the staff. The hospital staff, in turn, no less committed to sustaining its systems of meanings, values, and identities, must often turn to whatever tactics *it* can devise to maintain itself. The hospital, as an organization, may serve as a mechanism for sustaining those divisive perspectives which characterize the nature of human conduct everywhere. Thus, conflict and accommodation are recurrent motifs in studies of hospitals which stem from this theoretical point of view.

SPECIAL HOSPITALS—CRISES AND INVENTIVE SOCIAL INTERACTION

There are several sociological studies of patient-staff interactional patterns which serve to highlight the dynamic elements involved in the processes of conflict and accommodation. To a large extent such investigations have been conducted in "special" hospitals. These institutions are special for many reasons: They serve clients who are especially selected for care or treatment—perhaps because of their age, the critical nature of their disease, or the particular social characteristics upon which admission is contingent. Also, the organizational models deemed appropriate for general hospitals seem ill-suited to the conduct of work in special institutions. The proscriptions for professional behavior do not seem suited to those hospitals in which the illness is long or perhaps terminal. Further, the "line" worker may not be the physician himself but an ancillary medical person such as a physical therapist. The preferred relationship between patient and physician, between physician and hospital, and between patient and hospital are seldom found in special hospitals.

All these differences may be traceable to the pervasive lack of structure and the peculiarity of the work. As a consequence, roles are emergent and meanings ill-defined in these special hospitals. The interpersonal relationships between patients and staff are of preoccupying interest here as compared with general hospitals.

A Case of Hopelessness: The Incurable Illness. Fox's study of a metabolic ward is a case in point.[7] Patients in this hospital suffered from a variety of mysterious diseases about which very little was known. Indeed, the prime criterion for becoming a patient was that one had to be afflicted with a metabolic illness for which there was no known cure.

The uncertainties which marked the client problems transformed the typical doctor-patient relationship more commonly found in the focused crisis hospital. Specifically, the fact that the patients probably would not be returned to normal health made it ludicrous for them to "do what they could to get well."[8] While the patients were stricken with hopeless illness and the physicians with technical futility, these feelings were modulated by the strong personal ties which developed between the medical staff and the patients. Thus, the physicians found it difficult, even unreasonable, to maintain a posture of affective neutrality. This was inspired not only by the long period of time over which they interacted with their patients but also by the felt need to do for the patients on an interpersonal scope what the state of technology would not permit by a professional focus. The problems of the physicians were complicated by the fact that though cure might not be possible, the potentials for experimental research were tantalizing in their appeal. Although strong affectual ties might have developed between hospital staff and patients, the doctor was painfully aware of the fact that his client-friend might be even more seriously harmed by experimental manipulation. This hospital was special in that no fitting model of either appropriate patient conduct or professional conduct served as a reference.

Though the social structure of the metabolic hospital conformed in no way to that regarded as appropriate for the general hospital as a type of organization, it was a social order that had logic and meaning in its own right. And this meaning could be grasped only from an appreciation of the impossibility of cure engendered by the special nature of the disease entities involved.

Although the time period during which treatment occurs in special hospitals may be long and uncertain from the perspective of the objective observer, patients in these institutions seem capable of constructing a workable order of social time which is otherwise given in more general hospitals.[9] More important, client-constructed conceptions of time results in contingencies of organization which are not faced in other kinds of hospitals.

The Case of Indefinite Duration: Tuberculosis. Roth's study of a tuberculosis hospital takes as its point of departure the contention that since the disease is special, so too must be the interpersonal world in which tubercular patients must live.

Though the disease is specific, prognosis is not. Both physicians and patients are uncertain about the future course of the illness, the probability of its termination is quite certain though the date of its remission is not predictable. Thus, the tuberculosis patient seeks for clues to his fate—he tries to garner bits of information from patients more experienced than himself, from unwary nurses, and from doctors. These bits are then pieced together into a pattern of workable meaning which allows for the development of a patient world separate from that of the hospital officialdom. The staff, in turn, being equally caught up in the clinical uncertainties of the disease, attempt to withhold critical information from the patients, to give innocuous news and to project time in an indeterminant and ill-defined manner. As a consequence of the staff's inability to construct a set of workable meanings, the tubercular patient is thrust back to the company of his fellow-patients. They are at least more willing—if not more able—to provide the clues, the definitions, and the conceptions out of which the patient may devise symbolic order and temporal meaning.

The metabolic patients described by Fox and the patients observed by Roth are both special in requiring modifications of definitions of self, interpersonal relationships, professional guidelines, and organizational structure. The perspective taken by Fox implies that the symbolic dilemmas of the patients are at least partially resolved through the collaboration of patients with staff. From Roth's point of view, however, the patients achieve their own forms of accommodation in spite of the staff world.[10]

The Circumstance of Age: Children. Children present hospitals with yet another special contingency: Are the client materials too tender for the pressures which might be exerted upon them by a strict adherence to the professional mold and the application of the role of the sick? Or are they sufficiently pliable that they may be handled with impunity? Both options have precedence in medical organizations and the selection of either one importantly affects the content of the hospital system.

In a study of a psychiatric institution treating children under twelve years of age, Rosengren found that the hospital staff tended to fix upon the young age of their patients. In so doing they were reluctant to relate to them as "if they were sick."[11] Relationships between patients and staff acquired a personalized and informal nature, the character of which was reflected in the debureaucratized structure of authority in the institution. A diametrically opposed view is taken by Bettelheim who proclaimed that "love is not enough"—that superauthority not even befitting a general hospital is more appropriate for patients bearing the stigma of childhood. This definition of the selected client characteristic of age similarly informed the structural characteristics of the institution.[12]

Patient Restoration. The rehabilitation hospital is yet another institution which regards its work and its human materials as special.[13] It attempts two tasks which are in direct conflict with each other. This kind of hospital, which serves persons whose disablement is often massive, and by definition more or less permanent, tries at once to return the patient to his maximum capacity for social participation and to do what it can to see that the patient adjusts to the permanency of his fate. The rehabilitation hospital tries to return patients to the extra-hospital social world, but with the realization that this may not be possible the patient must also learn that colonization may be a more realistic goal.

Wessen's account leads to the conclusion that the problems, perspectives, and perceived tasks of the rehabilitation institution are *so* special that they may best be understood by conceiving of rehabilitation as a "social movement."[14] Conceiving of rehabilitation as a social movement suggests that the principal function of these hospitals is not the redefinition of meanings and symbols within the hospital context itself. They may serve in the carving out of a legitimate place in the social order for those persons regarded as worthy of such a place but who are incapable of fulfilling the places provided by the existing social structure. The hospital matrix is one in which the ideologies of humanism and technique are found in their most poignant coincidence—seeking for the vale of professionalism for those medical specialties regarded as strictly ancillary in general hospitals, and proselytizing for change in the extra-hospital community so that fruitful employment may be found on the basis of conviction rather than calculation.

The Terminal Case.   A mid-ground between staff-patient conflict and consensus is to be found in Glaser and Strauss' account of interaction in a terminal cancer ward.[15] It is here argued that patients and staff are seldom very certain about how much either knows, or ought to know, about what is happening or will happen. A situation of full consensus as elaborated by Fox is not likely to arise, nor is articulated conflict as reported by Roth a likely outcome. Rather, subtle forms of interactional confusion are likely to arise between patients and staff because one party to the staging may assume the other is privy to knowledge to which he in fact is not. The patient, for example, may believe that he is going to live; the nurse may know that he is going to die, but may assume that the patient is aware of impending death. The strains of the interactional context may be further aggravated by either the nurse or the patient (or both) making his assumptions openly known or trying to conceal his presumptions. Of course, conditions of presumed consensus may obtain for a while—only to be shattered later. In the mutual pretense context both patient and staff know that the disease is terminal, but both act as if this were not so. In such a situation, the interactional world in the hospital is one of carefully contrived disbelief, the real content of which must be carefully guarded and protected, lest its sad reality be revealed by an imprudent gesture, a mislaid chart, or an ineffectively coached student nurse. The hospital order, from such a perspective, is emergent, fragile, and continually shifting in rule and substance.[16] As Glaser and Strauss have said (and this is apparently true for most special hospitals), "we are cognizant of rules but are principally interested in analyzing interaction in terms of its open-ended and problematic character. Rather than focusing on interactional *stability* we shall be preoccupied . . . with *changes* that may occur during the course of interaction."[17] Just as the content of meaning and the conception of interactional reality for patients can be viewed as emergent and unstable from the symbolic interactionist perspective, so too can the structural aspects of the hospitals systems for the staff. Strauss and his colleagues correctly remind us that "the area of action covered directly by clearly enunciated rules is really very small."[18] The presence of mutiple professionals and quasi-professionals (especially in an institution such as Michael Reese's psychiatric unit) as well as participating bodies of clients demands that rules for conduct must be continually reassessed and negotiated. This is no less true for the ward-level personnel, such as attendants, who often feel that their day-to-day contact with the patients gives them special knowledge and license upon which to make up the rules as the work goes along. The patients, too, negotiate for privilege and exemption from the extant rules. This organizational responsiveness to the patient's expectations cannot help but result in continual shifts and variability in "hierarchical position and ideological commitments, as well as periodicities in the structure of ward relationships."[19]

THE PATIENT AS TARGET OR AGENT

While the focus on hospitals as bureaucracies emphasizes
the impact of structure—especially status and authority—on
the behavior of members, a focus on system or on interaction
highlights the view that pre-existing perceptions and structures modify activities in hospitals. It is no longer novel to
suggest that both patterns exist and themselves interact.
Considering now the impact of the perceptions of participants
upon hospital structure, it may be possible to pin down some
of the major problems involved through a more detailed
examination of studies of psychiatric hospitals.

In the "patient-centered" approach to psychiatric care are
found studies which express, in elemental and moving terms,
the helplessness and fragility of the human personality when
it finally succumbs to overwhelming stress. Paradoxically, in
reports about these humanitarian and enlightened institutions,
is found an equally dramatic demonstration that the persistent
demands of structure may not be ignored with impunity
even here. We focus now on the competing and conflicting
definitions which ascribe—sometimes to structure, sometimes
to perception—primacy in determining the forms and outcomes of institutional psychiatry.

Power Distribution and Patients. Whereas sociological studies
of other special hospitals have delineated the conditions of
role perception and meaning definition in the face of unique
contingencies involving "how much" of the patient shall be
treated, and for how long, studies of psychiatric institutions
yield a different set of themes.

A classic statement on psychiatric hospitals by Henry considers the effects that differential distribution of power between hospital units has upon decisions arrived at through
mechanisms of consensus. These effects seem to be the rule
in hospitals comprised of multiple units holding approximately

equal power, as in some elite psychiatric hospitals. Further, the smaller the number of "equal-power" units involved in decision-making, the greater is the likelihood that clinical decisions will be regarded as imperative and irreversible, as in some general hospitals. Some hospitals contain equally powerful units which perform similar or overlapping functions. In these cases the resulting lack of consensus probably besets the institution with persistent stress and conflict. Again, the case of the elite psychiatric hospital comes to mind as an example. Thus, stress and conflict, stemming from equal distribution of power, gives rise to a rich and volatile informal organization through which power is negotiated, with the possibility of transmitting organizational power to the patient group.[20] Where this condition is absent the patients are more likely to be insulated from the decision-making process as is typical in general hospitals.

The term "custodial" seems coincident with large state hospitals, while "elite" is nearly synonymous with small private establishments. What is retained in common in studies of these kinds of psychiatric hospitals is a focus on the nature of the work. Organizational structure and staff-patient interaction is considered as mainly supportive to the prevailing styles of work.

The Powerless Patient: Custodial Care. Goffman's study of St. Elizabeth's Hospital is perhaps the most representative of the first category, and especially in its picture of the repressive, dehumanizing, and brutal nature of work which presumably occurs in this kind of hospital.[21] Goffman confesses that he "entered the hospital with little respect for psychiatrists and left with even less."[22] Here the patient is stripped of his personal identity, imprisoned in both a physical and symbolic sense, humiliated by staff members who regard him not as ill but as crazy, and hazed unmercifully by other patients. The patient, frozen as he is into such a total institution, has as the only alternative to try to survive as best he can and to depart the place as untouched as possible by the experience. He may choose to rebel, and suffer even greater official retaliation. He may feign genuine insanity, and try thereby to garner some degree of sympathy and care from the staff. Or he may, in Caudill's terms, "live in the cracks of the hospital society" by carving out some measure of personal identity, worth, and autonomy.[23]

For our purposes, the principal point is that the functioning of such institutions is due largely to the ways patients are regarded and to the strategies of work which derive logically out of such a regard. Plainly, if patients are not thought to be fully human it is unlikely that they will be treated humanely. If their affliction is thought not tractable to modern science, then their hospitalization is likely to be little more than incarceration. In just such total institutions the ideology is one of punishment and coercion, and the organizational structure is similar to those found in prisons, concentration camps, and other places dealing with outcasts, recluses, and pariahs.

Less poignant though equally cogent are the studies by Belknap and Dunham and Weinberg.[24] Here, state hospital patients receive poor treatment not because they are unworthy, but merely because they are hapless victims of an inflexible government bureaucracy operating with too many administrative constraints and too few resources. It remains true, however, that treatment facilities *are* sometimes used to coerce. This situation may arise because of too few psychiatrists, too many work-hardened attendants, and the fact that hard-core psychotic patients fill the back wards, turning these hospitals into dumping grounds for the senile and the unwanted.

The sense of despair which accounts of state hospitals often convey may be traced to the fact that the logic of bureaucratic organizations requires that both patients and staff be devoid of "person" in order that the system remain orderly and predictable. The paradox has been noted by others and apparently is borne out in the case of some psychiatric hospitals. Bureaucracy, designed to function under the presumption of equality in the social context of democracy, lacks a capacity for individuated concern which accompanies the ethic of humanism.

If the trap of the total institution is a fundamental disregard for clients as persons, the state hospital may be marked by a structural incapacity to orient toward clients in any way not consistent with the value premises of the bureaucratic ethos. Studies of elite psychiatric institutions present quite a different picture in terms of both organizational structure and orientations toward clients.

The "Powerful" Patient. In addition to small size and private sponsorship, the elite hospital frequently bears the imprint of one person whose charisma diffuses throughout the organization and informs both its structural and operational aspects.[25]

The simplistic orientation toward patients—presumably the case in the large bureaucratic hospital—is less apparent in elite institutions. It is surprising, indeed, that the disavowal of customary criteria of patient evaluation, the elaboration of multiple treatment modes, and the addition of large numbers of professional and quasi-professional staff should lead so frequently to a less rather than a more bureaucratic form of organization. If the patient in the state hospital is regarded as ill to the point of becoming a nonperson, the deviancy of the elite patient may be regarded as so complex and inscrutable that he may not be regarded as ill in the traditional sense at all. The correlate seems also to be true: The staff member in the bureaucratic institution may personally acquire the infallibility which inheres in the organizational structure, but the worker in the elite institution may be fallible to the point of himself being regarded as ill and the patient as well.[26]

It would appear that in the bureaucratic hospital the worlds of staff and patient are sharply distinguishable and often marked by open conflict. But the distinction between patients and staff is modulated in the elite institution, so far in fact, that traditional conceptions of illness and organizational structure become irrelevancies.

A critical question is why this should be so. One answer is that the work orientations between clients and staff within the elite institution are remarkably similar to the conceptions, role sets, assumptions, and orientations which inform relationships between persons in the social order generally. On the other hand, the traditional hospital seems to emphasize the distinction between illness and normality. Perhaps because of this, the elite institution is more likely to have but thinly drawn boundaries. This is of critical importance for the types of relationships likely to develop *between* organizations, a point which will be explored in some depth in a later chapter. In any event, while the state hospital relates to patients as if they were ill or even evil, the posture of elite hospital stems from the assumption that patients remain persons in spite of their hospitalization.

Bockoven's account of the rise and fall of "moral treatment" is a classic statement of such a condition.[27] The sense of community presumed to have existed in the rural hinterlands of mid-nineteenth-century New England was mirrored in the small hospitals serving as protected places in which those who could not otherwise cope could be instructed in the arts of social living. These early psychiatric institutions attempted to duplicate the stresses, strains, and potentialities of the larger community without its sometimes cruel punishments for failure. As Bockoven writes:

> Charles Dickens' account of his visit to the Boston State Hospital in 1842 brings to light still more facets of hospital life

in the moral treatment era. He commented on the wide variety of activities available to patients including carriage rides in the open air, fishing and gardening and several kinds of indoor and outdoor games. Patients worked with sharp-edged tools and ate their meals with knives and forks. The patients organized themselves in a sewing circle which held weekly meetings and passed resolutions. They also attended dances which were held weekly. Dickens was particularly surprised with the self-respect which was inculcated and encouraged in the patients by the superintendent's attitude toward them. He made special note that the superintendent and his family dined with the patients and mixed among them as a matter of course.[28]

THE PARADOX AND INSTABILITY OF PERMISSIVENESS

The similarities between the old moral treatment centers and current conceptions of innovative psychiatric care are striking but it is historically the case that the decline of moral treatment occurred with population growth and demographic differentiation as well as rapid industrialization and urbanization. Such changes are not inconsistent with the breakdown of primary relations between patients and staff and increased bureaucratization of organizational systems in state hospitals. Moreover, the fall of moral treatment was accompanied by the rise of scientific psychiatry and the professionalization of the mental health occupations. These facts must be taken into account in understanding the more recent conception that institutionalized persons *are* tractable to specialized technologies and hence require treatment in organizations which are different from the social milieux in which "normals" interact. The prevailing preoccupation with interpersonal relationships and patterns of communication as distinctive features of the modern elite hospital has precedent in individual psychiatry, and is probably best represented in the well-known study of Chestnut Lodge, and in Caudill's study the *Psychiatric Hospital as a Small Society*.[29]

A discernible theme is a certain lack of clarity as to how patients are best handled and a corresponding awareness of the wide variety of stimuli to which patients are responsive. Hence, the main *tour de force* of such therapeutic communities are interpersonal relationships rather than a distinctive repertory of professional skills and techniques. Indeed, Hyde and his colleagues have gone so far as to contend:

> The important point here is that all personnel have full opportunity to grasp the implications of the simple truth that the professional members of the staff are operating on much the same footing as those who have had no scientific training.[30]

Structurally, the elite institution tends to be decentralized rather than hierarchical. Procedures are informal, rather poorly defined, and subject to contingencies. Role assignments for staff personnel tend to overlap formal professional distinctions. Finally, hospitals such as these tend to foster an "ethic of maximum communication" which serves at once to bolster a sagging *esprit de corps* often found in these hospitals and to preclude the development of an orderly and reliable internal structure.

The enthusiasm which greeted reports of some early experiments in milieu therapy was dissipated to a considerable extent by later accounts of the dysfunctions of total treatment hospitals.[31] As Rapaport and others have implied, the milieu treatment institution is rather thick on ideology but thin on technique. Consequently, there is a tendency toward "sloganeering" as well as some drift in organizational structure to more traditional forms and toward the selection of more specific and predictable technologies. Also, the expectation that all staff members should contribute equally to the therapeutic tasks places additional strain upon nonprofessionals, resulting in worker disillusionment and dissatisfaction.[32]

More to the point, are the results of a series of studies conducted by a team of social and behavioral scientists at the Columbus Psychiatric Institute and Hospital.[33] These investigations examined a key assumption underlying much of the argument accompanying the therapeutic milieu approach to psychotherapy: that even the most chronically ill, disoriented, and "back ward" mental patients are extremely sensitive to their environment. Of special interest is that the five wards of the hospital differed in a number of significant ways, and so approximated a "natural" experiment. The wards were different in the etiological viewpoints espoused, in the relative emphasis on and use of the various therapies, in the manner in which staff members were involved in the functioning of the ward, and in the attitudes of ward administrators and other personnel toward research and training. Differences were also found in the frequency of staff conduct, participation, and discussion at morning ward meetings.

The findings failed to show that the attitudes and psychiatric policies of key staff personnel significantly affect the ward behavior of mental patients. The overt behavior of patients seems to be only slightly affected by the practices of the unit to which they were assigned and in general is hardly distinguishable from that of patients in other units. Differences in patient behavior patterns were found, to be sure—but the greatest differences were associated with the sex, age, length of hospitalization, and diagnosis of the patients. A basic conclusion offered was that the specific characteristics of each psychiatric illness may be far more important in the determination of patient behavior than differences in unit substructures.

A NEW PERSPECTIVE: TECHNOLOGY DEFINES THE PATIENT

Hospitals and all other organizations are limited by the idea systems which inform what happens to patients, by the physical plants within which the work must take place, and by the equipment available to the hospital. This assertion gives rise to the argument that the way hospitals are organized and the fashion in which they define and handle their patients are both determined by the hospital's technological order.

Clients can be defined by organizations in many ways. A common contrast is between hospitals which regard their patients as "objects" subject to the routinization characterizing the processing of raw materials in industry, and those which view their patients as social beings who fully participate in the organization.[34] The place occupied by an organization along such a continuum will have important outcomes for the structure and dynamics of hospitals. If the industrial posture is taken, then the structures, supervisory strategies of control, and the manipulations of the factory arise as dominant. Patients will be approached *as if* their conduct contained no emotional content, and *as if* their lives contained neither a past, a socially relevant present, nor an organizationally significant future. Alternatively, if patients are defined by the organization as fully participating members of the society from which they come, then the hospital is likely to eschew the industrial model and accommodate itself to the fact that the client has been defined at once as normal but also deviant; as understandable but not completely knowable.[35]

As Perrow points out, some medical institutions have much the same technological imperative as does assembly-line production of automobiles.[36] Intake assessments in some psychiatric hospitals, diagnostic work-ups in general hospitals, and the sequence of events in obstetrical hospitals might typify the assembly-line medical technology. Rosengren and De-Vault have written:

> The normal circuit: admitting room, to prep room, to labor room, and finally to the lying-in room is adhered to scrupu-

lously. The physiological tempo would often indicate that at least one or more rooms might better be forgotten but the patient must adhere to this timing of movements from region to region, even if it means at a fast trot.[37]

Thus, the behavior of both patients and staff can be elicitated by the physical setting. It has been even more recently argued that what constitutes a viable organizational technology, and therefore the determinant of organizational structure and dynamics, is largely a matter of organizational option.[38] *If* the hospital officialdom believe that their technologies are predictable and reliable, then they will probably act toward their patients *as if* this were objectively the case, and probably by recourse to the bureaucratic model. If there is some doubt about the uniformity and predictability of the work to be done, however, it is more likely that a professional model of authority will be found.

As Thompson has pointed out, an organization may elect a "long-linked" operational philosophy out of which derives assembly-line procedures with their unique problems for both patients and staff.[39] Alternatively, an "intensive" technological posture may be found. Here there are no firm criteria specifying at what moment and in what sequence multiple technologies are to be activated. This is not infrequently the position adopted in some psychiatric hospitals, in some rehabilitation hospitals, and to a limited degree in some medical wards in general hospitals.

Perrow takes the position that *perceived* differences in the nature of the human materials worked upon leads to important differences in organizational structure.[40] One aspect of this theory is a continuum along which human materials are arrayed from well understood, to nonuniform and unstable. The elite psychiatric hospital might be located at the latter end of the continuum, and the custodial institution at the other.

In structural terms, the hospital which perceives its human

materials as being unstable and not well understood is likely to be characterized by a high degree of supervisory power and decision-making discretion and interdependence of work groups. Conversely, the hospital which perceives its working materials as stable and well understood is likely to contain more rigid and prescribed procedures for work with a lower degree of supervisory power, and by a minimum of interdependence of working units. Of primary importance here is the fact that this conception of organizations quite deliberately focuses upon the manner in which clients are perceived by the organization and its effect upon the internal structures and dynamics of hospitals.

Freidson's model is a perspective in this tradition. The importance of the degree to which the hospital imputes curability to the disease entity and the extent to which the sufferer is judged to be responsible for his own condition are stressed.[41] From this viewpoint, institutions which impute hopelessness or incurability to the conditions of their patients, are likely to resemble total institutions, with an emphasis upon containment and long-term incarceration. Those which impute curability to the disease are likely to contain more benign philosophies. The addition of the responsible—not responsible dimensions, however, yields at least four kinds of organizations as represented in Table 1.

TABLE 1

Modes of Managing Deviance by Imputation of Responsibility and Prognosis

Imputable Prognosis	Responsible	Not Responsible
Curable	Limited punishment	Treatment, education, or correction
Incurable	Execution, life imprisonment	Protective custody

Source: Eliot Freidson, "Disability as Social Deviance," in *Sociology and Rehabilitation*, M.B. Sussman, ed., Washington, Vocational Rehabilitation Administration, 1966, p. 77.

Organization judgments along both dimensions leads to the selection of different technologies for dealing with the persons and conditions so conceived. The first type, imputing both curability and responsibility, might be typified by the treatment of acute alcoholism and some communicable diseases. The second, involving curability with the absence of personal responsibility, is represented by the treatment of most illnesses in bureaucratically organized general hospitals. The third, incurability combined with personal responsibility, is probably best typified outside the world of medicine, though at times in history persons suffering from numerous afflictions were treated with this kind of impunity. Finally, incurablity combined with no personal responsibility is reflected in that form of benign care provided terminal cancer patients, some chronically ill persons, and geriatric cases. Freidson correctly points out that this scheme is especially useful in delineating the contrasting effects such differential definitions may have upon the social personality of the ill person. But it is equally important as a starting point in explaining how relationships between organizations and their clients may affect the internal structural characteristics of the defining hospital.

SUMMARY

According to social system analysis, hospitals are best understood by the fact that they must pursue goals which are occasionally in conflict—service and system maintenance. Also, hospitals must incorporate, in some degree, elements of all major institutional systems. Their complex organizational structures and dynamics represent this fact. Persons who work in or are served by hospitals can seldom be relied upon to act in ways which enhance the multiple goals of hospitals. They must therefore be induced to do so through the manipulation of rewards. The kinds of rewards and inducements used to integrate hospital staff members seem also to be related to the ways in which patients are manipulated and controlled. Invidious conceptions of superiority and inferiority cut across common-place notions of organizational structure and importantly affect the orderly progress of hospital work. Often patients expect different things from hospitals than what the organization is prepared to offer, and this gives rise to problems and dilemmas which are as yet unclearly understood.

In sum, the social system approach goes beyond bureaucracy by recognizing that hospital structure and dynamics need not conform in all respects to the classic conception of bureaucracy in order to be understandable. It goes further by explaining deviations from the bureaucratic model by turning to a more global and overarching theory of social action. In their most elegant representations, however, such explanations are seldom reduced to a level of concretion so as to provide an alternative theory of hospitals *qua* organizations, especially insofar as they contain participating clients.

If the social system approach goes beyond bureaucracy, the symbolic interactionists go within bureaucracy to the meanings implicit but not always self-evident in behavior. Structures are weak because for some participants they are virtually nonexistent. The hospital is here viewed merely as a stage upon which symbolic constructs, and the subcultures to which they give rise, become the strategy through which two disparate social orders are sustained. Consistent with the community morphology perspective, the hospital can be regarded as a mosaic of symbol systems held together by only the most tender of symbiotic ties. Hence, the organizational structures comprising hospitals of all kinds may not be the most salient reality which must be contended with, for they consist mainly of fragile linguistic constructs serving merely as vague conduct referents for the organizational participants. More important is the fact that these contrived meaning systems are, at root, fundamentally different for the staff and the clientele.

In contradistinction to the bureaucratic and social system approaches, the surprising observation is not that there is so little order and consistency in organizations, but really that there is quite so much.

The technological perspective is a recent development in the study of service organizations such as hospitals, and perhaps because of this it is not easily summarized. There are, however, those studies which regard the symbolic meaning of physical things in hospitals to be a limiting factor—leading either to assembly-line work processes or to "judgmental" procedures. There are those which regard medical technologies as determined by the perceptions which develop in organizations regarding the nature of the client population—thus presumably compelling different organizational strategies for handling them.

In spite of the remarkable mechanization of modern medicine, machine technology as an organizational ethic appears to be on the wane. This, in turn, is countered by the development of interpersonal strategies of persuasion with their consequent lack of certitude as to the responsiveness of the client to controlling efforts on the part of organizational authorities. On the one hand, the *machine technology* perspective presumes that the patient's sensitivity is mainly toward objects rather than to persons or symbols, and that the character of his response is told relatively easily in advance. On the other hand, the *person* oriented hospital makes the assumption that patients are more responsive to the social milieu than to the physical environment and that prediction of their conduct is more difficult—perhaps even impossible. In the case of the first technology, it seems reasonable to assume that a viable and persisting organizational structure can be devised, while the latter technology leads to unanticipated contingencies which call for more flexible and changeable organizational processes.

5

The Hospital and Its Environment

Hospitals obviously do not function *in vacuo*. They are imbedded in larger environmental systems which impinge in various ways upon them. This simple statement poses three problems.

First: How shall environmental systems be defined? Are they comprised of other hospitals which have the same or similar goals? Perhaps other types ought to be included, based upon the argument that goals are seldom reducible to the delivery of specific and generic services. Is it proper, even, that environmental systems be restricted to other *formal* organizations? Perhaps the concept should include *other* collectivities such as groups, publics, and institutional arrangements. Of first priority, then, is the need for a specific empirical referent which will allow for the demarcation of a relevant organization of organizations.

Second, delimiting environmental influence must focus on those features of the individual organizations which are being influenced or determined. The concept of influence has sometimes been used to explain the emergence of organizational goals, or internal structures, or styles of work, and other aspects of organizational life. A focus upon one while neglecting others, however, provides a truncated picture of hospital dynamics as they arise from extraorganizational forces.

Third, a key concern in interhospital analysis has to do with the strategies employed by individual organizations as they seek to cope with the problems engendered by external influences. These may vary depending upon the particular aspect of the organization exposed to external stress.

These questions are particularly relevant to understanding interorganizational relations among hospitals, and the larger medical care system of which they are a part.

DEFINING THE ENVIRONMENTAL SYSTEM

Community Morphology. The community morphology approach suggests that hospitals are in fact the products of external environments—of the ecological and demographic characteristics of the communities they serve. As a result, they ought to reflect some essential organizational features of the community and the larger sociocultural system from which they grew. In contrast to the social system point of view, the morphology approach seeks for detailed discriminations among a community's satellite organizations, each one of which is presumed to reflect the sector of the social structure it represents.

Not only are host communities critical to the patronage patterns of organizations—lending financial substance and differential prestige—they are also the reservoir from which both clients and staff are drawn. As communities differ in their socioeconomic composition and moral tone, so too will the structure of staff composition and patient population of the hospitals which they spawn.

Given the assumption that organizations can be neither more nor less than is the host environment, elaborately specialized medical complexes appear to be a product of differentiation prevalent only in metropolitan communities. Segregation by place also appears to be a unique capacity of high population density. A variant of this theme is that communities consist of congeries of influential persons who are in positions to effect, for good or for ill, the fate of their service organizations. This position takes the view that the organization of medical establishments is dependent largely upon their place in the informal power structure of the host community. Given ineffective or antagonistic relationships to the "powerful," hospitals must be economically impoverished and technologically ineffiecient at best, and subject to the worst ravages of goal displacement at worst.

The community morphology position arises out of the assumption that organizations stand in a state of unstable equilibrium with the sources of support, recruitment, and dialogue upon which they must depend. Such a condition may approach conflict—especially where the staff of such institutions is judged to be an improper reflection of the power system of the local community, and the clientele is viewed as residual and alienated from the otherwise orderly relationships which ought to inform linkages between hospitals and their community setting. The fate of the patient from the community morphology point of view has to be regarded as a by-product of the interface between organizations and the more significant and important publics in the community.

Interorganizational Analysis. A narrower, perhaps more sharply focused definition of the hospital's environment is the set of formal organizations with which it directly interacts. The state of interorganizational analysis as a field of study, however, is embryonic. There are few well-formulated conceptual frameworks and a paucity of empirical research. Notwithstanding the limited efforts at coping with interorganizational analysis, a fairly consistent theme can be discerned. This has to do with testing whether theoretical models designed to study the internal structure of organizations can also be of use in understanding interorganizational relationships. This matter is obviously of great importance in that the emerging problems of medical organizations seem to call for the development of new models of thought rather than more research to test the efficacy of older systems.

Although hospitals *are* the major treatment centers of the community and deserve intensive analysis, total health service is not rendered within separate hospital settings or in the offices of individual practitioners. "Complete" health is available only through networks of health agencies and organizations. Although these agencies vary in size, form, function, autonomy, and professional composition, they interact and comprise a health agency system serving the general community and the myriads of individual recipients.[1] Furthermore, the notion of a health agency system is in accord with the realities of recent medical events, innovations, and increasing challenges and demands:

> The changing morbidity picture, the growing philosophy of comprehensive care, the heightened efforts at decreasing in-patient hospital utilitization, and the gradual extension of health insurance to cover medical costs outside the hospital setting have combined to cause many hospitals to go beyond the mere provision of in-patient departments. Over the years, the services of out-patient departments have been broadened to include a wide range of diagnostic and therapeutic services to ambulatory patients in the general community. *The new functions assumed by the out-patient clinics have established them more firmly in a network of relationships with other hospitals and community agencies* (italics ours).[2]

As shown in Chapter 2, however, patterns of inter-hospital relationships, as well as the success or failure of such arrangements, differ greatly. Both style and effectiveness are determined not only by the availability of resources and the disease entities treated but also by the social class composition of the clientele group and the orientation of the individual agencies toward the clients selected for care. Thus, to say that hospitals are becoming more and more involved in *systems* of health care is virtually axiomatic.

Studies of "hospitals in context," then, may be grouped according to whether the observer's focus defines the environ-

ment as the total community or as a set of formal organizations which are in a critical relation to the hospital.

THE HOSPITAL AND COMMUNITY MORPHOLOGY

An early account of the association between the host community and the structural characteristics of its serving hospitals is found in Bockoven's history of moral treatment.[3] This
old form of humanistic care was in close contact with the
small New England communities in which relationships between patients, doctors, and attendants were but a mirror of
extra hospital commensalism. A reading of Bockoven's account
suggests also that the decline of community within the walls
of the moral treatment center was paralleled by a decline of
community outside them. Increased social differentiation of
the larger social order was accompanied by the rationalization, bureaucratization, and routinization of organization and
treatment in these hospitals.

A more contemporary example suggests that differentiations
marking community structure are mirrored—perhaps even refracted—in the hospital system, and that the power structure
of communities importantly underlie the kind and quality of
medical services abailable to patients. Belknap and Steinle
address this issue directly in their comparison of medical
care in Centralia and Watertown.[4] Although the two towns
were markedly similar in socioeconomic composition, Centralia's hospital system was second best as judged against
currently acceptable standards of hospital care: bed space
was crowded; less than half the available space was used
for diagnostic and treatment purposes; too much space was
used for waiting rooms, lunch counters, and other public
purposes; costs to paitents were too low to provide good
care; there were too few specialists on the staff; no social
services were available to patients; surgical standards were

minimal. The facilities in Watertown were in dramatic contrast.

The difference was traced not only to patterns of collective action characterizing the histories of the two communities but also to the present relationships between the hospitals and the local community power structure. High quality medical care was related to the integration of the hospital board members with the local community leaders. This in turn provided access to the several institutional spheres needed for mobilization for change and innovation in the hospitals. Indeed, the fact that the hospital in Centralia corresponded to the hierarchical and bureaucratic pattern typical of institutions constructed prior to the mid-1930s can hardly be understood aside from the fact that a viable and active community power structure exerting influence upon it vanished after that time.

The conclusion, precipitous but suggestive: In the absence of effective external systems, the presence of an integrated local community power structure seems essential for the maintenance of hospitals responsive to the increased demands for efficiency and broadly-based services now characteristic of the clients of modern hospitals.

Of special importance, however, is the fact that the hospital with strong associations with the community power clique delivered to patients not only technically more efficient care but a broader scope of services as well. It provided social services and family consultation as well as good medical care. The hospital which maintained but minimal links with the community "influentials" provided medical services only, and presumably not very good ones either.

A study of the hospital in its community context directly relevant to the social psychology of participant commitment is reported by Pfautz and Wilder.[5] This investigation of a small innovative psychiatric hospital revealed that indexes of *social* distance between categories of hospital members, patients included, was associated with indices of *spatial* distance from the hospital. Those of higher status in the hospital (board members, patrons and others with a demonstrated high degree of commitment to the aims and ideology of the hospital) lived close to the hospital. Those of lower status (nonprofessional workers and patients) with less of an investment in the hospital were drawn from a far-flung ecological base.

Professionals, however, deviated from this pattern. Although they were highly committed to the hospital, they lived far from it. One interpretation offered was that the cosmopolitan professional brings a different perspective to the hospital than do either the locally committed patrons and officers or the disengaged supportive personnel and patients. An inference of some importance can be drawn that both organizational structure and operational strategies designed to secure member commitment must contend with the fact that while hospitals may indeed be the products of the local community, this is not true for some staff members. In addition, such hospitals can probably expect less engagement from its patients than from those whose "property" it is.

A study conducted in upstate New York[6] revealed some dysfunctions resulting from too close an alliance between local community forces and hospitals. Specifically, the two hospitals which maintained close ties with the community influentials received much greater monetary support from the local community than did the two hospitals with weak community association. But the locally supported hospitals were disadvantaged in at least two ways. There always existed the possibility of unpredicted withdrawal of support for capricious reasons. More important, in terms of the contemporary medical scene, is that these two institutions received less support from available federal agencies and facilities. As Blankenship and Elling indicate, "Close alliances between an organization and a group which is external to it . . . appears to have potential disadvantages . . . there is always the possibility that the 'tail may begin to wag the dog.' In exchange for the currency and prerequisites of greater potential staying-power, the institution makes commitments which reduce its flexibility in other respects."[7]

Reliance upon local groups for support may carry with it these kinds of dangers; also, these patterns of support have been in the decline over the past half century. Whether this is due, as Schulze has suggested, to increased "nationalization" of community life, or to increased bureaucratization of the hospital as suggested by Perrow, must remain a moot point.[8] Whatever the cause, it seems clear that the increasing participation of the federal government in the health affairs of local communities further complicates the processes by which hospitals relate to external forces.

There is another important link between hospitals and the community—namely, clients and potential clients. Eliot Freidson, borrowing labels from Robert Redfield, characterizes the modern hospital as part of the great culture, while clients bear the lay culture.[9] Hospitals contend with a set of values toward health and norms for illness which may be in conflict with the standards of the modern medical setting. Of critical importance to the operation and survival of a hospital is its connection with the *lay* referral system through which potential clients often delay their appearance at a hospital or clinic: "We have seen that the first step in the history of a patient's complaint is self-diagnosis, followed by confirmation or alteration of the diagnosis when he consults others in his household. No further steps may be taken if the lay diagnosis so indicates and the complaint is bearable."[10]

The dilemmas of the modern hospital as they bear upon the lay culture of the client are apparently increasing, partially because innovations and modifications of the traditional hospital systems have required the inclusion of members of newly developed medical specialties. Not only do new medical specialists lack an established anchorage in the hospital structure itself, but they also have no traditional referral routes which tie them to clients. Hence, they are organizationally marginal and are subject, perhaps more than the standard physicians, to the vagaries of the informal client system in the community. As Freidson says, "Social work is a good example of such a new dependent profession, sustained by agents for the clients rather than by the client himself."[11] Although the newer medical professionals are "sustained" by others in their relations to clients, the substance of encounters between the innovators and the clients are of fundamental importance for the stability of the hospital.

THE GENERAL HOSPITAL AS A PARTICIPANT IN COMMUNITY MORPHOLOGY

General hospitals occupy an important place in the total medical system of a community, and especially so in the organization of the medical profession. They are the one place in which the modern physician can practice most efficiently with supportive equipment and a cadre of staff. Perhaps more important, they have been the most important avenue by which the aspiring physician can lay claim to a place of stature and prestige in the professional community. The wealthier and more prestigious the hospital, the more does affiliation with it result in enhanced professional status.

In addition, as community institutions, general hospitals normally arise in response to the needs and demands of a particular segment of the local population in an identifiable place in the community. Because of this, the aggregate of general hospitals in a city stands as a laboratory in which one can perceive some of the characteristics of the social structure of the entire community. Because general hospitals require support from the community, such institutions can be usefully exploited to elaborate the ways and degree to which the effectiveness of formal organizations can be informed by their place in the power structure of the local community. Finally, general hospitals are illustrative of the processes by which formal organizations seek autonomy, arising initially as the products of special interest groups in the community and tending ultimately to garner at least some degree of control over their internal affairs.

The role of the general hospital in the organization of the medical profession is no better illustrated than through Hall's study of the organization of medical careers.[12] Hall discovered that order and pattern could be discerned in the career routes traveled by young doctors. More important was the fact that these avenues to established professional status were intimately tied to the structure of the community and to its organizational personification in the hospital complex in the city. The importance of professional organization was observed in the fact that acceptance into medical school was often a result of sponsorship by a well-established physician in the community. While it is true that aspirants without such a patron did find their way into medical school, they did not attend prestigious schools.

A later career step was the securing of a residency in a "desirable" hospital. Hall found that this was most likely to occur in the case of young men sponsored by an eminent local physician (himself on the staff of the hospital) whose credentials bore the imprint of a prestigious medical school. Those who found their way into medicine without such sponsorship took their medical degrees in "second-run" medical schools, sometimes in foreign medical schools, especially in the case of young men from the ethnic communities of the city. If these doctors returned to their home communities, they usually did their residencies in the less opulent hospitals operating under ethnic or denominational sponsorship, and remained outside the central core of power and prestige in the professional organization and the community power structure at large.

The relationships between community organization, ecological structure, and hospital structure is further illustrated by Lieberson's more recent study of Chicago physicians.[13] Here the ecology of urban communities seems especially crucial to the medical profession—particularly for medical specialization, the class and ethnic characteristics of practitioners, and the social composition of clientele.[14] Some ethnically distinct physicians—especially Jews—tended to be more specialized than other physicians, to be located in the highly concentrated downtown areas of the city, and to draw their clientele from a wide socioeconomic range. Doctors with *other* distinct auxiliary characteristics—either lower class in origin or from more recently immigrated European groups—seemed to practice in regions separate from the city center. They drew their clients from more distinct populations in the community. The association between high differentiation of physician characteristics and client characteristics seems to hold up to a point. Beyond that, however, the structure of the metropolitan community seems able to accommodate a pattern of medical practice consistent with high population density—high specialization of service in conjunction with mass utilization.

At the same time, the cultural enclaves so often noted in urban settings may well mitigate against the realization of medical care programs designed to deliver services without regard to the social characteristics of either clients or practitioners. It has also been shown that the relationship between community structures and hospitals is to be observed in the degree to which hospital sponsorship affects the colleague context against which medical services are provided.[15] Lieberson, for example, found that physicians tended to hold appointments in hospitals the class and ethnic sponsorship of which corresponded to their own background. Consistent with Hall's earlier study, Catholic physicians predominated in Catholic hospitals, Protestants in Protestant hospitals, and Jews in Jewish hospitals. In addition, the Protestant hospitals in the city studied were the more prestigious, thereby providing their physicians with greater access to the informal professional community.

Of more importance, however, is the fact that each type of hospital tended to operate under different economic contingencies. This, in turn, informed the substance of the collegial relationships between doctors and, by implication, the posture of the hospital *vis-à-vis* the patients.

In confirmation of Hall's account, the elite medical system in the community was perpetuated by processes of membership selectivity and ritual induction in the Protestant hospitals. While the prestige and stature of a physician in an elite hospital was traceable to his informal position in the local medical community, status in the nonelite hospitals (more often operating under the economies of proprietorship) was gained by the physician's ability to mobilize a paying patient referral system upon which the survival of the institution depended. As Solomon points out:

> The nature of the relationship among colleagues is therefore quite different from what it is among doctors in elite Protestant hospitals, and, for the most part, doctors in other hospitals are not really colleagues at all, but rather, competitors who from time to time share a common interest.[16]

In general, the community morphology approach stems from the assumption that hospitals reflect the structures of the community in which they reside. The quality of hospital care seems traditionally to have been closely associated with the strength of link between the hospital and the influentials of the local community. While hospitals may initially arise out of community-wide demands for elite medical care, the outcome of organizational growth may be an alienation of the institution from the community and its domination by those who staff and administer it.

There is some evidence that power and authority are wrested not only from the community at large but also from the medical staff, residing finally in the administrative wing of hospitals.[17] According to Perrow's study, the successful mobilization of broad community support was followed by transfer of power from the Board of Trustees to the professional medical staff. This was traced to the increased technological specialization which successful community support made possible. Once the technical growth curve flattened, the critical issue became the allocation of resources within the hospital. Hence, the power of the technical-medical staff was diminished and that of the administrative personnel correspondingly enhanced.

We cannot say that such a power career is typical of all general hospitals, though it may occur with sufficient frequency to suggest that although the local community may give birth to hospitals, the institution ultimately achieves a degree of autonomy and specialization not originally intended. More recently, there has been some indication that the quality of medical service may be deleteriously affected by too well-established and inflexible ties to the local community. This shift may be accounted for by the massive programs in health and welfare which are often addressed directly to the hospital *system* in the community, circumventing the interstitial organizations heretofore central to a hospital's capacity to accommodate change and innovation. Finally, the client population potentially brings to the hospital a cultural content perhaps more consistent with the older forms of hospital organization than with more recently established innovations.

As a result of such community forces the fate of those served by general hospitals may ultimately be informed not by the values which gave rise to the organization, but by considerations administrative in tone and peculiar to the special place the hospital has carved out in the larger local medical community.

In all these perspectives toward the general hospital as a product of and participant in the community structure, however, the impact upon the patients remain unknown at worst and opaque at best.

INTERORGANIZATIONAL RELATIONSHIPS: PRACTICAL AND THEORETICAL PROBLEMS

Networks of organizations do exist—formally or otherwise—in systems of health care, but they remain largely unexamined. Modes of development, effectiveness, and future directions still appear either random or unknown.

There are several reasons for the lack of this kind of knowledge. Some are of a practical nature and have to do with the empirical realities confronting hospitals which daily have to *practice* their skills and utilize their organizational apparatus. The crisis orientation of the general hospital and its overriding emphasis upon specific technologies mitigate against the hospital's capacity to execute and assess medical care programs which differ in any radical way from traditional concerns with episodic illness intervention. The pressures of great numbers of persons seeking medical care—and the inaccessibility of the general practitioner in a mobile society—often means that the hospital suffers from acute personnel shortages. In many instances, shortage extends to standard resources: bed space, operating rooms, intensive care units, and emergency facilities.

Merely to keep abreast of accelerating demands and increasing costs of medical technologies strains resources to the limit in most cases. As a result, few resources, little energy, and perhaps even less imagination can be diverted to creative interorganizational planning. Considering these, it is not surprising that in many instances so-called affiliations and health agency networks are largely ad hoc arrangements among overworked and overburdened medical facilities, designed more in response to immediate crises and opportunities than to long-range objectives and probabilities. The scattered variations of interorganizational projects, their difference in scope and aims are best characterized as reactions to current and immediate environmental pressures and influences which have little allegiance to rational testing of effectiveness.

This is not to deny the viability of certain types of multi-agency relations. For example, the working arrangements between chronic illness hospitals and state and locally sponsored rehabilitation agencies, or the moderately successful experiencies of halfway houses for mental patients, may illustrate a responsiveness to current needs for newer organizational forms.

This brings us to another major reason for the dearth of guidelines for the developing interagency networks in the health field. We refer to the general lack of systematic knowledge about how to achieve effective interorganizational relations—whether involving health agencies or other institutions. Litwak and Hylton, for example, say that, "One major lacunae in current sociological study is research on interorganizational relations—studies which use organizations as their unit of analysis."[18] These authors refer to several attempts at such analysis and suggest that "little has been done in current sociological work to follow up the general problems of interorganizational analysis as compared to the problems of intraorganizational analysis, that is, studies in bureaucracy."[19] More recently Evan has noted that "Social science research on organizations has been concerned principally with *intra*organizational phenomena."[20] He goes on to suggest that "The relative neglect of *interorganizational* relations is all the more surprising in view of the fact that all formal organizations are embedded in an environment of other organizations as well as in a complex of norms, values, and collectivities of the society at large."[21]

It behooves us to examine some of the efforts at interorganizational analysis with a view toward identifying conceptual departure points and taking note of the relevance of these ideas for the problems of hospitals.

SCOPE AND LIMITATION OF THE INTER-ORGANIZATIONAL NETWORK

A critical question confronting interorganizational analysis is the issue of system ingredients—how large is the system and what are its component parts. Several illustrations point clearly to the conclusion that the scope as well as the elements are determined largely by the nature of the problem to which hospitals are separately addressed.

In the field of rehabilitation, for example, Wessen notes that:

> rehabilitation has not yet been crystallized into a typical organizational format. There is not yet an organizational pattern for rehabilitation which is typical of human activity in the sense that the school typifies education or the hospital the practice of medicine.[22]

Rehabilitation services are performed by a multitude of diverse agencies and institutions and delivered by a motley assortment of operatives and functionaries that very nearly defy traditional classifications. The over-all configuration, Wessen suggests, "is like a patchwork quilt, with both duplication and fragmentation of effort abounding."[23]

In the absence of clear organizational features by which to differentiate rehabilitation institutions from schools, hospitals, reformatories, nursing homes, prisons, and so forth, the problem of specifying system boundaries and potential interorganizational system membership is vexing. To meet this problem, Wessen suggests that it is useful to regard rehabilitation as a social movement—a social form designed:

> to elucidate . . . the relationship of formally or even functionally unrelated organizations to one another, much as the organization chart of a complex organization enables one to trace out certain relations of subunits to one another in terms of their relation to higher echelons of authority.[24]

A central problem for analysts in the fields of medical organizations is to determine whether an integrated system does exist or is in the making. If it is in the making, the guidelines for its orderly development are vague and the resulting final configuration is still largely in question.

A quite different focus regarding the nature and scope of an interorganizational system is reflected in Elling's account of how hospitals garner support in an urban community.[25] The major concern is with problems of coordination and cooperation among health and welfare organizations on the community level. Specifically, Elling describes how four hospitals attempt to plan for bed-space additions in their hospitals. Elling's analysis details the influence of the larger community in the failure to achieve the agreed-upon objectives. However, the attention paid to environmental influences such as religious groups, labor unions, the mass media, etc., is limited to their special relationships to key units involved; namely, the hospitals.

Elling's account sets forth some aspects of dynamic relations among a set of organizations and their environment. The main components of this system are the hospitals. Despite the range of important environmental influences, the interorganizational system remains "closed" because the hospitals are the focal organizations throughout the investigation.

Ranging somewhere between Wessen's open approach and Elling's closed interorganizational network is Levine and White's attempt to develop a conceptual framework for the analysis of the interrelations among various health and welfare organizations. These investigators dealt with twenty-two health organizations in a New England community. While the scope of that system appears well circumscribed, it does represent a considerably more diffuse field of study than that in Elling's report. Levine and White report, "Of the 22 health organizations or agencies studied, 14 were voluntary agencies, five were hospitals (three with out-patient clinics and two without), and three others were official agencies—health, welfare, and school."[26] In their attempt to conceptualize the nature of interorganizational relations, Levine and White delineate an organizational network on the assumption that the aims and commitments of the agencies involved *are* similar. They ought, therefore, on logical grounds to be more involved with each other than with other types of organizations. Hence the question whether a "true" system exists is a lesser concern than that of how organizations manage specific *problems* in their relation to other organizations. In other words, the *fact* of the existence of interorganizational networks can hardly be disputed; it is the substance of these networks that remains problematical.

In general, then, the scope and limitations of interorganizational systems appear markedly different depending on the problems posed and range from those investigations which regard the interorganizational network as problematic to those which assume that a system does exist. For the latter, the key issue has to do with the relationships between the parts.

RELEVANCE OF INTRAORGANIZATIONAL DYNAMICS

A second set of questions regarding interorganizational relations focuses on the internal features of organizations as they may affect external relationships. In a major contribution, Thompson and McEwen discuss interaction between organizations in terms of "goal-setting" processes.[27] They argue that the impact of environmental conditions upon individual organizations is manifested by a need to reappraise organizational goals and objectives.

Of special importance for understanding medical-welfare organizations is the contention that reappraisal of goals appears to be more difficult as the "product"—persons in these cases—becomes less tangible and less amenable to objective measurement. "In the complex society desired goals and the appropriate division of labor among large organizations is less self-evident than in a simpler, more homogeneous society. Purpose becomes a question to be decided rather than an obvious matter."[28] The strategic importance of goal setting for understanding the changing functions of hospitals and other health related institutions is obvious, though it can by no means remain the exclusive consideration.

Among the key issues hospitals confront as they relate to other hospitals is that of maintaining autonomy in decision making. In his discussion of the organization-set, Evan considers the importance of the size of the interorganizational network with which focal organizations must contend:[29] "A focal organization may have a relatively large or a relatively small number of elements in its set. Whether it interacts with few or with many organizations presumably has significant consequences for its internal structure and decision-making."[30] Evan hypothesizes that "the greater the size of the organization set, the lower the decision-making autonomy of the focal organization, provided that some elements in the set form an uncooperative coalition that controls resources essential to the function of the focal organization, or provided that an uncooperative single member of the set controls such resources."[31]

Decision-making power implies autonomy—the capacity to implement the decisions being made. The extent to which a hospital is free to exercise decision making will have repercussions for such important *intra*organizational factors as staff morale, ability to recruit staff and attract clients, and all those other organizational processes by which the needs of clients will be met.

In Wessen's discussion of the organizational problems of rehabilitation agencies, for example, it is noted that when hospitals are members of an "organization-set," the problems of autonomy and decision making become especially acute. The impact of the medical profession on rehabilitation and its personnel has been an unremitting source of irritation and has undeniably shaped the internal structure of rehabilitation agencies as well as the tenor of their goals and actual achievements to date.

A further illustration of the relevance of autonomy for the linking of organizations to their environment is provided by Levine and White. Their interest in organization domain is featured by a consideration of the extent to which organizations can effectively claim control of *future* goals: "The domain of an organization consists of the specific goals it wishes to pursue and the functions it undertakes in order to implement its goals. In operational terms, organizational domain in the health field refers to the claims that an organization stakes out for itself in terms of (1) diseases covered, (2) population served, and (3) services rendered."[32] Criteria of organizational efficiency, accreditation policies, allocation of both social and material resources, and other important aspects of internal structure are clearly related to the manner by which an organization resolves its domain problem. This, in turn, necessarily involves contact and negotiation with other organizations of the same type.

SUMMARY

Organizations serving health and medical needs, then, have problems of autonomy and cooperation similar to those faced by organizations providing other services to clients. Even hospitals with narrowly defined and immediate interests must make some concessions to environmental and social pressures in order to survive. Stated simply, hospitals always depend upon their environment for maintaining continuity of inputs and outputs. When the "product" is a service judged to be of very great societal importance—such as health—pressures for meeting social goals as well as organizational needs will correspondingly be greater. More important, these pressures will become even greater to the degree that needs are not satisfactorily met.

Whether or not a set of hospitals serving related needs must form an integrated system is of increased concern to the users as they become individually less able to coordinate their own use of the required services. A peak of frustration appears to have been reached in the field of health today, in that the organizations responsible for the dramatic specialization now characterizing what we call the medical system, have not yet altered the existing client referral system so that general access to the medical institutions will be available. Thus, whether a viable health care system does or does not exist, there is little doubt that it is now a functional necessity for the delivery of adequate service. Therefore, interorganizational analysis in the health field properly focuses on how organizations do in fact work together for common ends, and under what conditions such activity is likely to be enhanced. At the present *time,* however, there is but minimal interpenetration of this field of study by the more traditional conceptualizations which have informed the study of separate organizations.

PART THREE

THE CONTEMPORARY medical scene is in a great state of flux. Perhaps it is this fact which accounts for the many sociological studies of hospitals and patients during the past decade and a half. And sociologists have come to this task armed with an impressive conceptual and methodological armory. This is reflected to some degree in the wide-ranging studies reviewed in Part II.

The aim of Part III is to add to this conceptual armory in a way which is a step, perhaps even a short and halting one, toward integrating the three principal but usually separately pursued issues in the study of hospital and patients.

The classification of studies used in Part II is not wholly arbitrary. Indeed, studies of hospitals and patients seem logically to fall into three major categories: those which focus mainly upon the internal structural characteristics of hospitals; those which deal in social psychological terms with the patient as a person; those which deal with the hospital as but one unit among a larger set of units. All three are obviously of great practical importance for maximizing health care. In addition, the bureaucratic, social system, community morphology, and symbolic interactionist approaches have done good theoretical service and are likely to continue to do so.

What is offered in Part III is a way of looking at the hospital, the patient, and the medical system in a way which will keep the two neglected aspects at least in one's vision, while the third is highlighted.

Chapter 6 is concerned with the internal properties of hospitals as they may be affected by organizational definitions of patients. Chapter 7 looks at the conduct of the patient as he too may be influenced by the hospital's conceptions of its responsibilities. Chapter 8 deals with relations among groups of hospitals as they may arise out of the hospital's orientations toward its patients.

We do not pretend that this analytic scheme solves *all* the problems, either practically or conceptually. Nonetheless, key institutions and persons in medicine are today grappling with this monster, recognizing that a neglect of one member of this triumvirate—the hospital, the patient, or the system—is to invite disaster. Hence, we join the battle.

6

Hospitals and the Biographical
Career of the Patient

This review of the sociology of hospitals reveals a rich and varied literature. These studies focus on distinct problems and issues, some organizational and some interactional in scope. Moreover, one of four or five long-standing traditions underlie all of these efforts to frame an understanding of the contemporary hospital. As we have attempted to show, the use of one point of view leads to the neglect of elements that might be illuminated if a more synthesizing perspective were employed. Paradoxically, the great weakness of each point of departure and focus is its very analytic power—the capacity to elevate some aspect of the hospital world to a level of much importance and clarity, while failing to discern other equally important issues facing the modern hospital.

Here is posed the first of three problems: How to conceptualize hospitals and their patients so as to incorporate the strengths of these approaches less divisively than has been the case in the past. There are, in addition, two other problems faced by hospitals with which current conceptions of organizations seem unable to cope. The first is the increased responsiveness of hospitals to the strains put upon them by participating clients—their patients. The second involves the mounting pressures toward inter-hospital contact and collaboration. Thus, hospitals are confronted by three major problems: How to organize their work in ways best suited to meet patients' needs. How to react to the demands of a body of participating clients less easily subsumed within traditional "medical" models. How to relate to other organizations with similar or even identical purposes.

The remainder of this book is devoted to an exploration of one analytic model of organizations which may be useful especially for hospitals.

Many students of formal organizations, hospitals included, have shown increasing interest in the need to regard clients as critical facts in organizational life: Parsons states, "in the case of professional services there is another very important pattern where the recipient of the service becomes an operative member of the service—providing organization. . . . This taking of the customer *into* the organization has important implications for the nature of the organization."[1] Having made this point, the discussion turns to a systemic analysis of the ways organizations meet system maintenance requisites without pursuing this insight, the implications of which are not less true of hospital than of other client-organizations.

Blau and Scott point to some of the instances in which organizations might be understood in the light of client characteristics:

> It is perhaps a truism to say that organizations will reflect the characteristics of the publics they serve. A technical high school differs in predictable ways from a college preparatory school, and an upper middle class church is unlike the mission church of the same denomination in the slums. While such differences seem to be important and pervasive, there has been little attempt to relate client characteristics systematically to organizational structures.[2]

It is obvious that patients present hospitals with a wide range of characteristics for involvement and control: the specific disease in its limited organic aspects, the social etiology from which it sprang, the family setting to which the recovered patient must return, the psychological make-up of the patient as its bears upon his capacity to withstand hospital treatment and to cope with post-hospital adjustment.

Other patient characteristics may be incorporated into the hospital. *Any* specific patient characteristics may have an impact upon the hospital, and even *more so* when such a characteristic is regarded as relevant by the hospital and deliberately taken account of.

As a matter fact, hospitals selectively define those patient characteristics thought to be salient for the purposes of the organization. Perrow, for example, argues that hospitals belong to that class of organization which attempts to alter the state of human material—such material being self-activating, subject to a multitude of orientations, "encrusted with cultural definitions,"[3] and embodying a wide range or organizational relevancies.

The importance of organizational definitions of people for the internal structures has also been emphasized by Etzioni. A key determining factor for him is the confrontation between service to clients as an *ideology* and as an instrument of manipulation and control.[4] Specific to hospitals, the implication is that the medical care delivered to patients can hardly be understood without a careful consideration of what the "service" accomplishes for the hospital as an organizational system seeking control, stability, and continuity of its external relationships.

Another conception of the interface between clients and organizations is found in Eisenstadt's discussion of debureaucratization: If the client is perceived as a scarce resource upon which organizational survival depends, "The more [the organization] will have to develop techniques of communication and additional services to retain the clientele in spheres which are not directly relevant to its main goals."[5] In other words, when hospitals are in a competitive relationship with other organizations providing similar services, a typical response is to broaden or enrich the services offered in order to attract more patients. This can be accomplished either by offering "better" medical service in depth or by addressing the "whole person."

Finally, the symbolic interactionist tradition is reflected in the work of Glaser and Strauss. Their paradigm of *awareness contexts* is useful in explaining the interpersonal contingencies of being ill and dying in a hospital. Patients and staff must often interact on the basis of contrasting knowledge of what is occurring and of conflicting definitions of the situation. Speaking about the paucity of studies which are concerned jointly with organizational structure and social interaction, they conclude, "in so much writing about interaction there has been much neglect or incomplete handling of *relationships* between social structure and interaction that we have no fear of placing too much emphasis upon those relationships. . . . The course of interaction may partly change the social structure within which interaction occurs (italics ours)."[6] And the larger the number of patient characteristics taken into the hospital, the more complete interpersonal relations become.

Thus, there is consensus around the fact that patients are important participants in hospitals, but the descriptive character of the materials leading to this consensus has precluded a realization of their points of convergence and of their analytic potential.

A PERSPECTIVE TOWARD PATIENTS AND HOSPITALS

In spite of the divergent observations which have been made concerning patients and hospitals, a major theme is discernible. That theme can be expressed by saying that organizations such as hospitals attempt to intervene in various ways in the "biographical careers" of their patients—that is, hospitals may attempt to intervene in the present and future life of their patients with varying scope and in varying intensity. In so doing, hospitals must be organized internally so as to effect this intervention. They must also contend with the various interactional contexts to which differential intervention leads. They also must confront other hospitals in their community environment with the limitations imposed by their orientation toward *their* patients.

The delivery of a "service" such as health care to clients implies that hospitals must intervene in the human career of their patients. In so doing, they attempt to make an imprint upon the kind of person the patient will be, both now and later in his life.

A strict definition of what the client's biographical career means shall not be set forth just now. This failure is subsumed under Dilthey's famous dictum that "We always understand more than we know." We can do no better than to use Everett C. Hughes' words:

> Every man is born, lives, and dies in historic time. As he runs through the life-cycle characteristic of our species, each phase of it joins with events in the world. . . . Such joining of man's life with events, large and small, are his unique career, and give him many of his personal problems . . . one's ambitions and accomplishments in turn, involve some sequence of relations to organized life.[7]

Hence, while one's life is shaped by the rituals, occasions, and systems of etiquette that are the cultural reservoir of the society, it is also molded by the many formal organizations to which persons become attached for varying periods during a lifetime. And just as the human career may extend in both time and space, the nature of organizational intervention may also vary along these two axes.

A hospital's interest in the careers of its patients may range from a highly truncated span of time—as in the emergency room of a general hospital—to a nearly indeterminate span of time, as in a long-term psychiatric facility, chronic illness hospital, or tuberculosis sanatorium. In whatever case, the hospital's resources, arrangements for work, and relations to its environment are informed by the orientation the institution has in the patient's future course of life and especially for the retention of organizational power over the patient once he has physically departed the confines of the institution.

There is a second kind of client intervention. Here the client is viewed in terms not of biographical time but of biographical space. That is, hospitals may have an interest in but a limited aspect of the patient as a product of and participant in society. Again, the short-term general hospital comes to mind as an example. Others may opt for a broader scope of interest in the patients, as in the case of pychiatric outpatient clinics or some rehabilitation agencies for the blind. In these, the total person is incorporated into the hospital system and worked upon assiduously.

In sum, the *longitudinal* patient career extends in social time, but the *lateral* dimension extends in social space. Hospitals, however, may attempt to intervene in either of these two aspects of the human career—broadly or specifically in the present, and in the short or long haul. That is, lateral or longitudinal intervention may vary independently of one other.

In fact, there are four kinds of orientations, each of which has significantly different consequences for work in hospitals, the substance of hospital life as it unfolds on a day-to-day basis, and for the hospital's relations to its external environment. These variants are depicted in Table 2.

Such a system implies that certain similarities are to be found in hospitals which have a similar lateral interest in their patients' lives, even though they might differ sharply in the extent of their longitudinal concern. One would expect to find some similarities between a general hospital and a tuberculosis hospital, even though the latter has a long-term interest in the patient's biography. The orientation of both hospitals is highly specific and focused upon well-defined

TABLE 2

Organizations and the Client Biography

Empirical Examples	*Biographical Interest*	
	Lateral (social space)	Longitudinal (social time)
Acute General Hospital, Emergency Room	—	—
TB Hospital, Rehabilitation Hospital, Public Health Department, Medical School	—	+
Short-Term Therapeutic Psychiatric Hospital	+	—
Long-Term Therapeutic Hospital, Some Chronic Illness Hospitals	+	+

and technologically accessible disease entities. Although each may well take account of additional factors such as occupation, family life, age, sex, and so forth, the relevancy of those to the defined patient problem is either minimal or given a low priority in the hospital.

By the same token, hospitals which have a similar stake in the future life of their patients should have some features in common despite the fact that they may differ markedly along the lateral dimension. For example, a long-term psychiatric hospital should resemble in some aspects a tuberculosis hospital, even though the former may have a broad interest in the patient as a person.

The remainder of this chapter shall be devoted to exploring some of the implications of the client biography perspective for hospital organization, as tentatively supported by empirical studies of hospitals.

THE PATIENT BIOGRAPHY
AND ISSUES OF COMPLIANCY

One persistent problem in hospitals has to do with the strategies which render patients tractable to the internal needs of the organization.[8] The four types of client biographical interests outlined here give rise to different kinds of patient control problems and to different arrangements for achieving compliancy.

It is useful to make the distinction between *conformity* and *commitment* as modes of compliancy. Each requires different conduct on the part of patients and results in different strategies for achieving compliancy in the hospital.

In the case of compliancy through conformity, assuring patients' adherence to conduct rules is the key problem. However, the investment of the patient in the ideology of the hospital is more at issue when commitment is desired. The broader the hospital's interest in the patient's life-space, the larger the number of conduct alternatives on the part of the patient regarded as organizationally relevant. One important consequence of problematic conduct conformity is a large investment of staff time and effort in determining relevant rules for conduct and in devising strategies for enforcing them. In extreme cases, this may lead to a reliance upon "control" expertise in the hospital, in which the distinction between clean work (service) and dirty work (control) becomes blurred, and the service ideology is informed by the need for control. One study of these problems in psychiatric hospitals for children argues:

> . . . even a *sub-rosa* concern for order and conduct conformity . . . leads to the routinization of procedures for handling those problems; it becomes a part of the administrative and policy system in its own right. Thus, the means by which containment is enforced . . . often becomes so particularized, routinized, and the task so repeatedly distributed to particularly "skilled" persons . . . that it becomes a profession in the institution and a value in itself.[9]

Conversely, hospitals with a more focused interest in their patients are likely to be those in which the conformity of patients to rules is of lesser importance. In some cases, conformity may be regarded as given and therefore unproblematic. This may occur either because of the physical layout of the hospital (isolation wards and private rooms) or by the physical incapacitation of the patient (e.g., quadraplegics in rehabilitation hospitals), and also by the dynamics of the patient subculture which may itself mitigate against patient misbehavior.

In the long-term hospital, however, the compliancy problem is different because the commitment to the patient's future biography may extend beyond the time when he will be physically present in the hospital. Here, rearrangement of the patient's life cannot be accomplished merely by manipulation or the exercise of coercion when the patient is on the grounds. On the contrary, patient compliancy is best achieved by getting him to believe in either the moral goodness or practical fitness of the future the hospital attempts to shape for him.

The compliancy problem, therefore, is here attacked by transmitting an elaborate ideology to the patient so that self-control may be exercised once he departs the institutional housing. Thus, while the patient in a medically oriented psychiatric hospital is not expected to believe in or understand the theoretical grounds upon which the use of electroshock therapy rests, the patient in a psychoanalytically oriented hospital may experience a profound transformation because of the symbol systems to which he has been exposed.

A central difference between the long and short-term hospital is that in the former the patient is expected to *control himself* as a consequence of the strategies of commitment to which he has been exposed; in the latter, he is expected to conform in his post-hospital life only insofar as enough was done *to* him while he was a hospital patient. The fact that the long-term hospital must devise mechanisms for "checking-up" on the efficacy of the resocialization of its departed clients stands as a clue to some of the consequences of long-term inter-organizational relationships in the health field. The laterally oriented hospital, however, is forced to impose a wide scope of conduct rules which must then be accommodated to its ethic of service.

In terms of the client biography model, patterns of conformity and commitment take the shape as indicated in Table 3.

TABLE 3

Orientations toward Clients		Compliance Problems	
Lateral	Longitudinal	Conformity	Commitment
—	—	no	no
+	+	yes	yes
—	+	no	yes
+	—	yes	no

Contrasting problems of patient compliancy—deriving from differential investments in the careers of patients—give rise to different types of problems for hospitals which are attended to by contrasting methods of resolution.

PATIENT BIOGRAPHIES AND PROBLEMS OF STAFF CONSENSUS

The nature of a hospital's concern with the patient also gives rise to contrasting problems of consensus among the staff. A persisting dispute in hospitals has to do with whether agreement exists as to what work shall be done and how it should be accomplished. Organizations may confront this contingency in either of two ways. Conflict may be recognized and acted upon so that its resolution is given a formal place in the social structure of the hospital. Conflict may, on the other hand, be relegated to the informal system of bargain and negotiation. As far as these distinctions are concerned, the patterns indicated in Table 4 are likely to occur.

TABLE 4

Orientations toward Clients		Consensus Difficulties about	
Lateral	Longitudinal	Means	Ends
—	—	no	no
+	+	yes	yes
—	+	no	yes
+	—	yes	no

In the typical short-term general hospital, for example, the specificity of orientation toward patients results in clear priorities as to the importance of different occupational skills in the quick repair job to be done. There is little basis upon which competitive processes can emerge to be incorporated in the officially sanctioned system of work. This finely graded system of status is reflected in nearly every sphere of activity in such a hospital, including the norms which guide interaction in the surgical team, permissible expression of humor among the staff, the adherence of staff members to official aseptic rules, and ceremonial standards governing the ways in which staff members of varying rank come together to constitute a working team.[10]

The specificity of orientation characterizing this kind of hospital, as well as the instant removal of the patient, implies little need to devise criteria or mechanisms for evaluating long-term outcome, or the allocation of hospital resources for this purpose. Nor is there any need to establish limits to longitudinal responsibility. In fact, the reverse is often the case: pressures exist to get the patient out quickly rather than to elongate his tenure.

Kramer's study of a day-care psychiatric center illustrates this point:

> The question soon arises in the mind of either patient or staff as to whether the time for leaving the unit has been reached. Though there is no rigid rule concerning length of stay, staff feels internal and external pressure about persons who are "staying too long." Internal pressure comes from the intensive treatment philosophy. . . . External forces operate in the form of pressures for turnover; new admissions to be accommodated, waiting lists to be reduced.[11]

This does not mean that stress and strain do not occur in the highly focused "quick" hospital, only that it is seldom subject to formal procedures. Conflict occurs at the informal and extra-institutional level: claims for status are made by those whose place in the hierarchy of professional priorities is somewhere other than at the top.[12] Power alignments develop among staff involving agreement of a *quid pro quo* type. But on the whole, structured competition for priority is blocked by the presumption of *rank inequality* which exists at both the operational and administrative levels.

At the same time, this kind of hospital is subject to pressures from the outside to take the whole person into account rather than some specific part of him, and to intervene in the patient's life for a longer period of time. Considering the short-term general hospital as the archetype of the community institution, it is easy to see that its technical elegance and elaborate cadre of ancillary personnel lead to periodic interfaces with its "publics," which attempt to alter the hospital's existing priorities. Substantively, if the bane of the general hospital is the accusation that physicians are technically competent but often without human feeling, the cross borne by the more broadly oriented hospital is that while general medicine may be well-meaning, its humane edifice rests upon a weak technological foundation.

Similar counterpressures are to be expected in terms of the

hospital's intervention in the future life of the patient. Thus, the long-term tuberculosis hospital must somehow cope with the patient's contention that he is retained as hospital property for too long. However, the short-term general hospital is often accused of discharging patients before they are fully recovered.

Quite the reverse pattern is typical in the broadly oriented and long-term institution. Here is to be found greater formal response to the presence of conflict. In view of the felt need for official consensus regarding means and ends, such a hospital continually contrives official and new devices for dealing with conflict resolution. While it may be true that the initial roots of conflict may arise out of the informal system of power alignment and personal negotiation, these issues are swiftly made subject to formal methods of solution. Here is to be found a proliferation of systems of communication, specialized staff and team meetings, and repeated attempts to develop a consistent and coordinate medical technology.[13] The not infrequent outcome is a continual reorganization of systems of authority and decision making, continual addition of staff members with finely discriminated skills and techniques—all with an aim to resolving problems of technology coordination and staff conflict. In sum, the lateral and long-term hospital involves a changing formal system of authority with a staff conflict culture, the content of which is continually co-opted into the formal system of the hospital.

PATIENT ORIENTATIONS AND THE
SHAPE OF HOSPITAL AUTHORITY

The breadth of intervention in the patient's life space will have important consequences for the structure of authority within the operative or medical worker line, while the extent of intervention in the patient's future life course more closely affects administrative authority.

In the general hospital, for example, the specific and short-term orientations will be accompanied by "pine-tree" forms of authority in both the operative and administrative lines. Conversely, broad and long-term interests in the patient's life will lead to dual "oak-tree" structures as represented in Table 5.[14]

TABLE 5

Orientations toward Clients		Patterns of Authority	
Lateral	Longitudinal	Administrative	Operative
−	−	△	△
+	+	▽	▽
−	+	△	▽
+	−	▽	△

In contrast to the debureaucratized oak-tree pattern, one feature of pine-tree authority is a capacity for clarity and decisiveness in decision making "at the top." Here the hierarchical pattern of authority renders decision making smooth, easy, and utterly understandable and acceptable to subordinates.

Coser has pointed out some of the consequences of these differences as observed on both a surgical and a medical ward:

> the line of communication on the medical floor is clear-cut and follows a scalar system, decision-making there generally proceeds through consensus. On the surgical floor, however, where the line of communication is not strictly adhered to, authority is not, as might be expected, diffused and shared, but tends to be concentrated and *arbitrary*, with decisions proceeding by fiat from the visiting doctor or the chief resident.[15]

Jules Henry also has noted some of the problems connected with each kind of authority system, and especially how the oak-tree pattern arises out of a broad concern with the patient's life space:

> One can see how readily a system of multiple subordination (*oak tree*) comes into being . . . a large number of tasks must be performed on each patient . . . hospital tasks are numerous, frequently unrelated to each other, and characterized at times in addition by the quality of *emergency*. The tasks are said to be unrelated because, for example, there is no relationship between seeing that a patient does not lose his false teeth and giving him psychotherapy. Yet the same nurse is sometimes supposed to do just that.[16]

In the typical general hospital, the specificity of intervention in the patient's present and future life leads to a dominant technological core around which a priority of occupational skills can be devised. Moreover, task assignments are likely to be so highly differentiated that the line worker—the nurse as an example—has little difficulty in locating her place in the over-all operation. Hence, this pattern of authority results in formalized rules for conduct which are more or less easy to follow. As Coser says:

> the surgical (*oak tree*) and medical (*pine tree*) wards were directly across the hall from each other. Walking from one to the other . . . one would notice immediately a superficial difference in the atmosphere; joking as well as cursing, laughing as well as grumbling could be heard at the surgical nurses' station. . . . On the medical ward the atmosphere seemed much more "polite." Joking or cursing there was an exception; informal talk between doctors and nurses was rare.[17]

Finally, Henry and others have pointed to yet a further important consequence of oak-tree structures for hospitals; namely, staff dissatisfaction at the lower levels:

> the organizational structure was not considered satisfactory by the personnel; the data showed much agreement that it was difficult to work in the system, that there was a problem of definition of function, and that information did not "behave" as it should.[18]

Differences in orientations toward the patient's life not only result in these kinds of authority patterns in hospital, they also call for the presence of different kinds of professional and occupational representatives in order to complete the desired work.

PATIENT ORIENTATIONS AND STAFFING SHAPE

When work is defined in different ways, it demands the presence of persons with different kinds of skills and of varying degree of professional stature. Often when full professionals are not available, less talented and less trained people are elevated to professional status in a hospital and expected to do this work. More generally, however, variations in the hospital's efforts to alter the present and future life course of patients results in differing proportions of professional and administrative personnel (see Table 6).[19]

TABLE 6

Orientations toward Clients		Proportions of Staff Components	
Lateral	Longitudinal	Professional	Administrative
—	—	small	small
+	+	large	large
—	+	small	large
+	—	large	small

A short-term commitment to the patient means that only a few highly specialized administrative tasks have to be accomplished. This is in distinction to the situation in long-term hospitals, where a larger administrative *cadre* is needed to maintain records and to seek out, codify, and nurture contact with *departed* patients.

By virtue of the short period of time for which patients are the responsibility of general hospitals, administrative tasks are well focused and routinized, requiring a small number of "officer" status personnel, and a correspondingly larger number of clerks, stenographers, medical secretaries, and so forth.

Administrative patterns in the long-term hospital are likely to be quite the reverse. Work here is not subject to routinization, but contains many of the elements of policy-making. It is, therefore, more frequently implemented by staff personnel rather than clerks.

Similar patterns will be the case among the *operational* contingents in hospitals. That is, specificity of orientation will lead to a comparatively small, though organizationally powerful, professional medical staff. Specificity of focus implies that the hospital's work rests upon an articulated technology, the implementation of which requires that work be organized around a single professional group whose "property" the technology is: physicians in general hospitals, psychiatrists in psychiatric hospitals, physical therapists in rehabilitation hospitals, and so forth. Moreover, the medical technology used in such a hospital is not the exclusive product, property, or domain of the specific hospital in which it is practiced. Rather, it stems from and belongs to a far-flung professional and scientific community. This fact has implications for the audience to which different types of hospitals address themselves, and more importantly for the professional "social types" it attracts and rewards.[20] This small but conspicuous professional staff in the specifically focused hospital is supported by a correspondingly larger number of ancillary personnel whose skills are selected and differentially rewarded on the basis of their presumed contribution to the main professional skill.

A broad interest in the patient's life is likely to weaken the dominance of any particular medical group, through the employment of a large variety of semiprofessionals who are awarded at least the accolade of equal status and responsibility. This process may, in extreme cases, lead to the domination of the operative activities of the hospital by lower level semi- or even nonprofessionals.[21] Cooperation by lower level workers can occur especially when the hospital is economically pinched, as in the case of many state psychiatric hospitals which attempt to treat the whole person without a corresponding increase in resources. The dysfunctions of this "professionalization of nearly everyone" have been pointed out many times:

> [The situation] . . . is more likely to involve a decrease in professional orientation toward patients and an increase in more diffuse, generalized interest among persons. Even the accouterments of professional identity may be lacking among the staff—nurses without uniforms, lab technicians without white coats, and doctors without stethoscopes. . . .[22]

The pseudo-professionalization characteristically occurring on the heels of a broad orientation toward the client's life space can and does have profound effects upon hospital policy in general and the degree to which novel and creative innovations in medical care emerge.

This is perhaps no better illustrated than by the following:

> The desired end of such a meeting of minds is that it be on the common ground of investing energy in learning. On this basis, personnel can come to understand that Milieu Rehabilitation is not a matter of a professional person applying his knowledge and having orders carried out, but that it is a research enterprise every step of the way with every client. Viewed from this perspective, *personnel are in no way providing purely ancillary services in the usual sense* . . . they are research workers whose powers of observation, thoughts, and communication are vitally important (italics ours).[23]

In contrast to the more specifically focused hospital, this kind is more likely to construct a special rationalization as well as a unique *modus operandi*. It is, in short, strong on ideology but weak on technique. This difference in the technological equipment of hospitals has important consequences for the introduction of innovations in the organization.

PATIENT BIOGRAPHIES AND INNOVATIONS IN HOSPITALS

Hospitals may innovate in either of two ways. They may introduce *technological* changes such as new mechanical equipment, new ways to increase organizational efficiency, reduction of time-cost formulae, more accurate criteria for evaluating work production, and the like. By way of contrast, hospitals may innovate at the *ideological* level. The development of new rationalizations, novel conceptions of the "meaning" of the work being done, alternate ideas to justify goals, and variations in cause and effect ideas are here involved.

It is suggested that a hospital's capacity to innovate in each of these ways is closely related to the previously outlined organizational structures, which themselves derive from the hospital's orientations toward the patient. Specifically, it is proposed that innovation occurs as shown in Table 7.

TABLE 7

Orientations toward Clients		Susceptibility to Innovation	
Lateral	Longitudinal	Technical	Ideological
—	—	yes	no
+	+	no	yes
—	+	yes	yes
+	—	no	no

In the specifically focused hospital the presence of a selected and well-articulated technological core makes it possible for the institution to *add to this* repertory in an additive sense as improvements. Indeed, the longer and more salient this additive process becomes, the less such a hospital is able to turn away from its highly focused orientation, reverse its course, and adopt a broadly based orientation toward its patients. The more elaborate and sophisticated the medical technology becomes, the less it will be seen as resting upon whatever ideological backdrop may have originally led to its establishment. In general, the more specifically focused a hospital becomes, the greater is its propensity to accommodate technological innovations which are *consistent* with, and can be rationally integrated with, that which it already contains. This may partially account for the oft-noted difficulties in attaching *functionally* meaningful social or psychiatric service departments in general hospitals, as well as for making the distinction between care and cure in general hospitals organizationally cogent. Perhaps most important (and an issue to be pursued in a later chapter) is that this kind of hospital —because of the ease with which it innovates at the technical level—becomes increasingly less capable of turning away from its original goals in order to pursue new ones.

This kind of "quick-repair"–"quick-release" hospital is but minimally susceptible to ideological innovation. The lack of a long-term engagement with the patient means that such an organization has little contact with all those other, perhaps differentially committed, organizations which may later be responsible for the future career of the patient. As a result, it has few occasions to take part in the dialogue of multiple organizations-in-contact, which can often be the source of reassessments of the aims and meanings of work. Because the patient's reorganized life is seen as satisfactorily accomplished through the application of a relatively specific technology, such changes can quite easily be thought of as separate from, and certainly not dependant upon, a coordinate ideological foundation. The specifically focused and short-term institution can be that which best embodies the process of cultural lag as found in organizations: dramatic advances in technological repertory combined with an ideological framework perhaps more relevant to an earlier era.

The more broadly focused and long-term hospital stands

as a contrasting type, subject as it is to a great deal of ideological turmoil and a minimum of technological innovation. Such an institution contains a multiplicity of technologies and, as a result, the central organizational problem is that of coordination rather than addition. In fact, the coordination problem may often be met by strategies of consensus-building —itself leading to ideological change.

More important is the fact that this type of hospital— committed as it is to a long-term intervention in the patient's future—must encounter a rich variety of *other* organizations (real or implied) with different technological cores and of contrasting ideological persuasion. An important outcome of this contact and communication is a rich interchange of ideas and arguments, which ultimately must have their impact upon the long-term hospital.

We mention only briefly a third type of hospital—the specifically focused *and* long-term institution subject to *both* technological and ideological foment. The rehabilitation hospital may well exemplify such a pattern. Here the operatives and administrators each sponsor a different form of innovation and change, and must often face each other in conflict as to which shall have priority. The conflict centers on which shall take precedence—the changing conception of the "mission" of the hospital as it may influence the long-term social welfare of the patient, or an increase in the hospital's machine technology. Such institutions may be suspended in a state of continual crisis and dilemma, with the patients as the most alienated of participants—confused about the hospital's claims for technological efficiency and its appeals for self-transformation.

This discussion relates to yet a further issue; namely, the patterning of decision making about patients and the pacing of the flow of work.

PATIENT BIOGRAPHIES AND WORK RHYTHMS IN HOSPITALS

It is useful to make the distinction between *judgmental* and *imperative* decisions, and between *rapid* and *slow* work tempos. By imperative is meant those decisions regarded as inescapable, and compelled by forces and processes not reducible to persuasive strategies. These kinds of decisions about patients are ones in which the human being serves merely as the articulating agent or vehicle transmitting the decision to others so that its irreversible outcome may be implemented. Judgmental decisions are quite different: they are created out of interaction and communication, and hence have a tentative quality about them. In contrast to imperative decisions, these *are* reversible and permit of numerous alternatives. In short, imperative decisions have a "thing-like" quality, while judgmental decisions are more nearly the product of symbolic constructs.

The distinction between rapid and slow is also one of degree. Work in some hospitals is done much faster than is work in others. In some hospials one aspect of the treatment process follows more or less instantly upon the heels of earlier parts: a surgical sequence as compared with psychoanalysis is a case in point.

The manner by which decision making and work tempos relate to the hospital's orientation toward the client's life is shown in Table 8.

The specificity of orientation in the general hospital, for example, combined as it is with a highly articulated division of labor, is often accompanied by the development of *sequential patterns* of work. Here, one activity must await the completion of a prior state. However subtly, the activation of stage *B* is contingent upon the empirical facts signaling the completion of stage *A*.[24] Thus, the decision maker must be sensitive to the criteria which compel the work to move on

TABLE 8

Orientations toward Clients		Work Rhythms	
Lateral	Longitudinal	Decision Making	Work Tempos
−	−	imperative	rapid
+	+	judgmental	slow
−	+	imperative	slow
+	−	judgmental	rapid

to the next stage, rather than direct himself to the readiness of other workers to express their agreement with the decision. Both patients and staff are in some sense carried along by external forces which they can direct but cannot reverse.

In the case of the obstetrical hospital, for example, work does have this sequential and imperative character:

> The normal circuit: admitting room, to prep room, to labor room, to delivery room, to recovery room and finally to the lying-in room is adhered to scrupulously. Timing may also be disturbed if key personnel happen to be absent from one of the places in the timing sequence. One evening, for example, a man rushed into the service claiming that his wife was about to have her child and that no one was in the admitting office. The doctor's advice—in all candor and sincerity—was that she was probably in false labor, and then encouraged the man to return to the admitting room.[25]

The same generic pattern holds for administrative activities in the short-term hospital: admission, securing of insurance policy numbers, recording of expended hospital resources, totaling of fees, exacting payment, and discharge of the patient. All of these constitute imperative decisions stemming from the specificity of orientation toward the patient's life space as well as from the clearly marked time period involved. The relatively rapid tempo is obvious—the quicker one stage is complete, the more rapidly will the next impress itself upon the transmitter. Whether the hospital's concern with the patient *really* extends for two days or two years, the significant point is the sense of urgency about the work.

Sometimes, indeed, the rapid pace of work in such specifically focused hospitals can produce what the objective observer can regard only as macabre practices. Mechanic, in referring to Sudnow's study of the handling of death in two different hospitals writes:

> He illustrates in various ways how the handling of the dying patient may reflect the needs of the staff to cope with their work, even at the cost of committing significant improprieties. Sudnow, for example observed a nurse trying to force a woman's eyelids closed before she died because it would be more difficult to do so after she had died. . . . On a busy ward, where death is a frequent occurrence, the wrapping for the morgue may be started while the patient is still alive.[26]

Events such as this involving time moving in advance of itself is characteristic of the highly focused and short-term hospital in which the social structures of decision making and work rhythms seem to outstrip the more naturally expected series of physiological events. In the obstetrical hospital previously referred to, for example, it was observed that:

> lack of a natural tempo seemed to be handled in a number of ways in order to impose a "functional" tempo where a "physiological" tempo did not exist. . . . In the delivery room itself, there seemed to be an attempt to impose a tempo—to adhere to a pace of scrubbing, of administering anesthesia, and so forth. There was also emphasis upon keeping track of the length of time involved in each delivery. . . . The "correct" tempo becomes a matter of status competition and a measure of professional adeptness. The use of forceps is also a means by which the tempo is maintained in the delivery room, and they are so often used that the procedure is regarded as *normal* (italics ours).[27]

Perhaps the most dramatic view of the crisis atmosphere which prevails in this type of hospital can be observed in the postmortem investigations into why the elaborate machine technology failed. These often acquire the tone of a juridical investigation, with the implication that some failed to "read" the imperative clues, or acted too slowly after having read them. But the weekly staff conferences in the elite psychiatric hospital communicate little of this sense of urgency and technical breakdown.

They more often resemble reflective and academically modeled seminars attempting to construct some degree of meaning out of the inscrutable mysteries of the complexities of a whole human person—past, present, and future:

> Once a week there is a core staff meeting, frequently attended by interested professionals from other sections of the hospital, in which *any problems* may be discussed. . . . Thus the meetings serve the dual functions of intra- and inter-staff communication and problem solving. The content of these meetings varies considerably and includes such items as acting-out behavior, depression, admission of a new patient, how to raise a patient's level of activity, whether a patient's upset is due to his therapists's going on vacation, should a patient be encouraged to look for a job in the community . . .(italics ours).[28]

Of course the broadly oriented and long-term hospital *is* the most contrasting type. In comparision with the mechanistic criteria for decision making of the general hospital, a particularistic stance toward patients is possible here. This stems from the fact that the hospital is faced with a technology coordination problem—in which the relative weights given to each social medical intervention can be tailored to each case. Sequential activities are seldom found. Simple cause and effect assertions are seldom the basis of action. In short, imperatives are absent.

As a result decisions are made less on the basis of irrefutable fact, but more on the strength of plausible argument. In extreme cases, the root of decisions is not the nature of observation of the patient, but more the unfolding of interpersonal relationships among staff members—the outcome of the human relations approach to supervision—the latent roles of some members, or the charisma of one person.[29]

In addition, there is not the sense of urgency so characteristic of the short-term hospital. Events need not occur over night. There is time to reflect, to ruminate, and to come to considered judgments. The pace of work is slow, stages of progression for patients are elongated, and movement between each stage is hardly perceptible. The patient is gradually coaxed and induced through the hospital, rather than marched in an orderly sequence through it. This last point, how patients are inducted into and are passed through hospitals, is deserving of more detailed consideration from the point of view of the client biography perspective.

7

The Patient in the Context
of the Hospital

> The conception of the model physician contains, by implica-
> tion, clues as to the nature of the model patient . . . there are
> conceptions of the ideal patient: about what is wrong with
> him, about his social and economic characteristics, about his
> acceptance of the physician's authority and prescriptions, his
> understanding, his cooperation and his gratitude.
>
> EVERETT HUGHES, "The Making of a Physician"

Everett Hughes' words are true also of the need for hospitals to induct their clients into the organization in ways consistent with what it will try to do to their personal career.
Individual staff members—because of their more powerful
positions—obviously contribute in a marked way to the induction of the client. But even they have to be dealt with so that
they will contribute to the chosen organizational intervention
in the patient's biographical career. Thus, the content of
social interaction in hospitals consists partially of the residue
which follows efforts to induce both patients and staff to
adhere to the desired organizational orientation. We consider
here only the first matter: the induction of the client so as
to make him a proper patient.

Drawing upon Merton's classic distinction (and as we have
upon his visual representation), Rosow makes the distinction
between socialization for value change and for alterations in
behavior.[1] This scheme asserts that variations in socialization

along these two dimensions—if successful—will produce four social types. Each has a distinctly different impact upon the permanence of the organizational system under conditions of both crisis and quietude. Rosow's framework is reproduced in Table 9.

TABLE 9

Forms of Socialization

Socialization Types	Adoption of	
	Values	Behavior
Socialized	+	+
Dilettante	+	−
Chameleon	−	+
Unsocialized	−	−

The *unsocialized* patient escapes an inductive experience quite untouched. He remains the same in what he does and what he thinks. He is a genuine "pilgrim passing through" who takes little from the experience and contributes nothing to it.

The *socialized* patient, however, is transformed most perfectly. He thinks of himself differently than he did before. He acts differently too. The salience of the experience may be so great at the "value" level that he becomes troublesome in the hospital precisely because it has such deep meaning for him. That is, not only does he take much from the induction experience in terms of act and attitude, but he also has the capacity to contribute to it. The *dilettante* is produced by that experience imposing superficial behavior change without fundamental changes in values: A fair weather friend not to be counted on in times of crisis. Finally, the *chameleon's* overt activity is pliable, though his basic values are sustained intact. He is, nonetheless, a reliable person to have about in moments of crisis. He has the capacity to act in required ways, however fleetingly. The danger, of course, is that he may bring to bear upon the situation irrelevant values or behavior patterns more suitable elsewhere.

The main point is that hospitals, by virtue of their chosen intervention in the client's career, may inadvertently produce these types of patients. We suggest that organizational socialization takes the form seen in Table 10.

TABLE 10

Client Biographies and Social Types of Clients

Orientations toward Clients		Socialization to		Patient Type
Lateral	Longitudinal	Values	Behavior	
—	—	no	no	unsocialized
+	+	yes	yes	socialized
—	+	yes	no	dilettante
+	—	no	yes	chameleon

Once more the patient in the general hospital typifies the lack of induction characteristic of this type of organization. The fact that the patient may not be psychologically prepared to act the unsocialized role stands as a clue to some of the fears and apprehensions about hospitalization frequently noted in studies of hospital patients. These fears often remain subterranean in the general hospital, revealed only in the privacy of conversation between the patient and his visitors. At the same time, the increased awareness on the part of hospitals of the frequent desire of the patient to be "instructed" about hospital life in order that his fears may be allayed, suggests that as a consequence of trying to induct the patient more effectively, hospitals may, inadvertently transform their more basic orientations toward their patients.

Patienthood in the short-term—quick-repair hospital, however, simply does *not* constitute patient induction. Fear-provoking as this might be for many patients, the unsocialized *is* functional for the general hospital inasmuch as the organizational system need not depend very heavily upon his voluntary contributions to the system, nor can the unsocialized play much of a disruptive role in moments of crisis. We may say only parenthetically, that just as the general hospital does not induct its clients, neither does it *"out*-duct" them. Never having socialized the initial raw material, the hospital need not concern itself with desocializing the finished product.

As pointed out earlier, much attention is paid in the lateral hospital to insure the patient's adherence to the rules of the organization. Here the induction process is likely to be long and intensive, with graded statuses demarking neophytes from those having traveled farther along the way to full membership. This may also be noted by insignia of patient-rank, ceremonies which signify passage from one rank to another, with systems of review which pass upon the appropriateness of the patients' condition and attitudes justifying elevation to more complete membership. There are, in fact, structural evidences of this as in the case of multiple staff meetings and clinical review teams in the elite psychiatric hospitals and tuberculosis hospitals, and consensually validated professional concepts by which the process is given pseudo-empirical reality. Patients may resist identification or they may be in the "countertransference" stage.[2] Given the fact that socialization is a dual process—conducted partially by the hospital officialdom and partially by more experienced patients—much power lies in the hands of patients themselves. Hence, relationships between patients and staff do not have the "command" quality that they do in the general hospital, but are more negotiative in nature.

Finally, induction in the broadly oriented long-term hospital involves *both* behavior and value aspects. As a result, issues of patient *control* are seldom easily separated from those of achieving ideological commitment: Efforts to maintain behavior compliance are frequently phrased in moral or ethical terms, thus attacking *both* requirements at the same time. This coincidence of behavioral and value control sometimes can have profound effects, even upon the strategies employed to govern relationships between staff members. As Blau and Scott report:

> In certain types of service organizations, such as casework agencies and mental hospitals, pseudo-democracy often takes the form of a therapy-oriented or psychiatric approach to supervision. In this approach the subordinate is not blamed for imperfections in his performance or for failing to conform to directives; instead, his behavior is analyzed to detect what unconscious forces have led to his resistance. . . . *What is conceived to be a very democratic method of supervision —not blaming subordinates but helping them understand their problems—turns easily into a manipulative controlling device* (italics ours).[3]

This dual commitment to behavior change and ideological engagement may well account for what Perrow has said to be contrasting viewpoints informing the conduct of staff toward patients in elite hospitals: "administration-centered" versus "patient-centered" standards.[4] Administration-centered criteria demand adherence to policy, order, quietude, lack of disagreement, and restriction of patients' movements phrased in the name of "security." Patient-centered standards, however, emphasize spontaneity, creativity, originality, freedom for the patient, and patient self-expression.

As contradictory as these may seem on the surface, and as confusing as they may be to the patient, there is no inconsistency given the fact that such a hospital must induce *both* behavior conformity and ideological transformation—the first accomplished through administration-centered tactics, the second by patient-centered devices.

Not only must this kind of hospital induct its patient, it must "out-duct" them as well. That is, the patient must be returned sufficiently altered as to retain the imprint of the hospital, but adequately desocialized so as to function normally in the larger community. Often, out-duction processes call for the design of special intermediary institutions—out-patient clinics, day-care centers, half-way houses, and so forth. These, too, have the same problem as does the parent hospital in severing the elongated tie which has been achieved between the hospital and the patient. The reluctance with which departure from such intermediary institutions occurs is well illustrated by Landy and Greenblatt's account of the Rutland Half-Way House:

> The ties that bind the resident to the House are not easily severed. . . . While some residents were not pleased with the idea of leaving the House, indicating that they probably found life there preferable to be in the community, many were able to effect their own discharge in agreement with the director.[5]

More frequently, however, and due partially to the great costs involved in maintaining these intermediary hospitals— out-duction is taken over by separate organizations in the community: visiting nurses associations, after-care programs in the local community, private practitioners, and so forth.

Whatever the tactic employed, the career of the patient in this kind of hospital is, if not long by the calendar, psychologically elongated with stages of progression which change slowly though inexorably.

Patients in hospitals face yet a further problem having to do with how they are initially brought into the institution and take part in its special culture.

PATIENT BIOGRAPHIES AND ROLES FOR PATIENTS IN HOSPITALS

In a very thoughtful and suggestive essay, Wheeler has pointed out:

When a person moves into a new institutional setting, a major problem he faces is understanding the setting and coming to terms with its demands. He must develop a workable "definition of the situation" to guide his action. . . . The socializing agents will have their version of this process, but since he is a recruit and they are not, his position will be different.[6]

The manner by which a new patient carves out a place for himself in a hospital derives mainly from whether other persons have preceded him there and have communicated to him a workable definition which he can copy. Four socialization contexts are outlined by Wheeler (see Table 11).

TABLE 11

Social Context of Entering Members

	Individual	Collective
Disjunctive	TYPE I Oldest child in family; first occupant of newly created job	TYPE II Summer training institute; group of visiting scholars in foreign country
Serial	TYPE III New occupant of a job previously occupied by another person	TYPE IV Schools; universities; professional training centers (approximated by prisons and mental hospitals)

Patients entering disjunctive-individual hospitals must, quite literally, make a place in them anew each time. No role model is provided, nor is there a prior-patient-cohort to aid the newcomer in becoming a member. This is obviously most often the case in hospitals like the short-term general hospital. Patient induction is even more lonely and disjunctive in the accident room. In these hospitals, the patient may carry with him only the lore concerning hospitals and illness which he has drawn from the cultural reservoirs of society. The degree to which lower-class obstetrical patients are especially prone to approach hospitalization against a backdrop of lore and superstition has been described:

> A lack of formal education and with extended kinship ties with grandmothers and great-aunts as lifelong agents of socialization—it seems more reasonable that she [the lower class woman] should act out the anxiety she has over her "illness," not in the context of the doctor-patient relationship, but rather within the framework of her own lower-class subculture. Part of that subculture consists of a body of lore and superstition to which persons turn in the face of personal crises—not unlike the ways in which groups sometimes turn to bizarre and incredible ideologies which also deny the "real world" when faced with a perceived collective calamity . . . the blue-collar woman is [likely to face] *her* personal crisis by means of a resort to that body of lore and belief which is an indigenous part of the subculture from which she comes.[7]

Hence, movement into the patient role may be more the product of "dame rumor" than of either instruction or rite of passage.

There is no readily available etiquette as to what conduct is appropriate for the *ex-patients* of the highly focused and short-term institution. Despite the trauma—both physical and psychological—the patient may have suffered while resident there, no post-hospitalization structures exist through which the experience may be collectively reviewed and given meaning, and therefore understanding and forgiveness. This is true especially in the case of patients who have undergone alterations which subsequently distinguish them markedly from other persons in the community. MacGregor, for example, tells of a young woman who underwent radical facial surgery:

> Until her operation, Charlotte had been a very social and outgoing person. She enjoyed herself and other people, loved to dance and play bridge with friends. Now she refused to go anywhere. "I couldn't stand the staring." She had a "steady" boyfriend, but would no longer go anywhere in public with him. She refused to meet new people because "it made me so nervous and self-conscious." . . . She refused to see anyone after office hours, preferring to remain alone in her room and listen to the radio.[8]

This of course is an extreme example, but it is used to illustrate the point that former patients of institutions such as the general hospital can seldom collectively share their medical experience with others. The experience *was* disjunctive, therefore the ex-patient must cope with it on his own later.

The situation in the serial-collective institution—the laterally oriented and long-term hospital for example—is quite the reverse. The broad scope of intervention and the length of time for which the hospital's imprint is intended means that the new patient enters a fully socializing organization containing rather clear avenues of induction into the ways of the hospital. The patient enters a hospital which presents him with a rich variety and broad range of alternative roles, made visible to him by both word and deed, and he is induced to adopt any one of these.

Moreover, patients leaving this kind of hospital become organizational ambassadors in a very real sense, and thus are capable of passing on to others the fundamentals of appropriate conduct there, and even to retain some measure of association and contact with the hospital. Landy and Greenblatt, for example, express this result in describing the typical reaction of former patients of Rutland Half Way House:

> Thus, the transitional function of the House does not termi-

nate with discharge, but tapers off gradually until the women have reached the stage, once in the community, when all their relationships are with "outsiders;" . . . It is as expectable for the former resident to continue to visit the House as for the former soldier to consort with his "buddies" in a veteran's organization, or for the former student to join his alumni association.[9]

As useful as this form of induction may be for maintaining the stability of the hospital system, it can be quite disruptive when, for whatever reason, the hospital undergoes stress and strain. As Wheeler points out:

The serial pattern, precisely because of its stability, risks stagnation and is likely to be undesirable from the point of view of agents when things are going badly. There is the likelihood that the former recruits will train the new ones using the defeating pattern. Should morale be low, older members introduce the newer ones into the low morale system. Should lower level persons be disrupting the program, they are likely to attempt to indoctrinate the new recruits with their viewpoint.[10]

Whatever problems are engendered by the serial and collective induction processes which take place in the broadly oriented and long-term hospital, it is also true that the patient— once he has departed—can never quite recapture his pre-hospital self. The experience he has undergone cannot help but have far-reaching implications for his social personality. As Goffman writes concerning the former patient of just such a hospital:

While some roles can be re-established by the inmate if and when he returns to the world, it is plain that other losses are irrevocable and may be painfully experienced as such . . . certain roles are lost to him by virtue of the barrier that separates him from the outside world. . . .[11]

Thus, in some hospitals the patient's future biography is rather permanently fixed by events that occur during the course of hospitalization. Socialization of the patient in some hospitals has a tradition with the members of each new cohort formed in the image of the old. This is essentially what Wheeler means by serial pattern. In others, patient induction and the subculture to which it leads arise out of the processes of collective behavior and meaning definition as each new patient cohort manufactures it anew. Roth's account of how tuberculosis patients construct workable conceptions of time during their hospitalization is illustrative of this pattern:

> Career lines may be divided between those where each participant starts running as soon as he comes to the track (continuous system) and those where the participants have to wait for a bunch to collect before starting off (cohort system). . . . Only the draftee army and the school system use a cohort system. With this system there can be no doubt what the appropriate reference group is for measuring one's progress—one starts off and travels with the same group all the way. With a continuous belt . . . it is not so clear who one's closest colleagues are. . . . The participant must not only "dope out" the nature and sequence of the bench marks; he must also construct an appropriate sub-group from among his potential colleagues to serve as a primary model for his own career expectations . . . .[12]

Patient induction in *most* hospitals leads to a round of interaction within the confines of the hospital which is volatile, emergent, and fraught with *collectively shared uncertainty.*[13]

It is clear that different patterns of patient socialization (either to values or to behavior) and the alternate contexts of patient induction to which they are related are likely to produce quite different kinds of patient subcultures in hospitals. We now turn to this matter.

PATIENT CAREERS AND HOSPITAL SUBCULTURES

Two aspects of patient life which are of much importance to hospitals are (1) whether the behavior of patients is basically in conflict with or in accommodation to the demands of the hospital system, and (2) whether the prevailing patterns of conflict or accommodation are of collective and organized types, or are more individual in nature. Depending upon the hospital's orientation toward its patients, we suggest that patterns of patient subcultures take the basic forms as shown in Table 12.

TABLE 12

Orientations toward Clients		Nature of Conflict	Subculture Pattern
Lateral	Longitudinal		
—	—	accommodative	individual
+	+	conflict	organized
—	+	accommodative	organized
+	—	conflict	individual

Again, the general hospital comes to mind as a clear example of the first type. Remembering that this kind of hospital makes little effort to "socialize" its patients in either a value or behavioral sense and also that the general hospital patient is inducted in a "continuous belt" fashion, it is then understandable that the patient never has full access to the hospital's social structure. He is, to be sure, a participant in it in ways already suggested. But he affects it by virtue of the manner by which he has been perceived and defined by the hospital; he never acquires *control* over his own impact.

The fact that this kind of hospital has a specific and short-term interest in the patient has added importance because every patient is especially addressed—each in a somewhat different way. It is this slight difference in patient individuation which partially accounts for the absence of an ongoing and viable patient subculture.

Lacking as they do a basis for interaction and consensus,

patients in the typical general hospital must confront the institution during the course of their residency quite alone, getting neither support nor approval from their colleagues. Paraphrasing Moustakas' touching account of the death of a mother in a hospital, the patient here "lives within the infinite loneliness of the unique."[14] This is not to say that the patient in the "lonely" quick-repair hospital may not undergo much the same kind of self-transformation as happens in the broadly focused and long-term hospital. The difference, of course, is that it occurs as private disclosure rather than through shared awareness. Quoting Moustakas again, the hospital which fails to make a place for a patient subculture cannot help but produce inadvertently "the gripping, painful, exhilarating, and beautiful experience of being utterly alone and separated from others."[15]

By reason of its specific focus, this kind of hospital offers little opportunity for an organized subculture to develop among the patients. Also, it provides few occasions on which patients may interact with one another in ways unrelated to the established aims of the hospital. The hospital solarium is still a lonely place. Isolation of patients from one another can be furthered by the physical accouterments of privacy in the general hospital. In the labor rooms, for example, curtains quite effectively deny patients access to one another, and therefore to the entire web of social relationships in the hospital.[16] All of this means that patients in the general hospital are powerless *vis-à-vis* the hospital officialdom; they can muster no united front. Save for the extreme tactic of "discharge against medical advice" (which occurs infrequently) the patient can do little more than devise his own private ways of coping with the demands of the hospital.[17]

Patterns of patient subculture are very different in the hospital which attempts to intervene broadly in the patients' life space and for a very long time. The broad scope of control which the hospital attempts to maintain over patients leads quite naturally to conflict patterns. This, combined with the long-term effort to fashion an alternate future biography for the patients, renders the conflict subculture a collectively shared one. We do not mean that conflict necessarily takes the form of open hostility on the part of patients, but merely that the patients are likely to counter the norms, definitions, and meanings which emanate from the staff with their *own* conceptions to guide them through the hospital. The hospital, in turn, attempts to get the patient to accept its official prescriptions. Ordered patient conflict is represented in how the following patterns among patients differ from the "official" ones:

> The patients, however, accept conventional euphemisms for mental disorder, such as "I was overworked and overactive, so I became nervous and needed a rest." "I was in need of a rest and was run down, so I was put in the hospital."[18]

The hospital, of course, has its own words to describe the events and problems precipitating illness. Again, the hospital may place a patient's personal possessions in safekeeping, but the patient may respond: "What's going to happen to my things while they're denied me? They are going to be destroyed by some other attendant who doesn't know what she's doing. They are going to be appropriated by this one and that one."[19]

Patients frequently learn to disguise their real feelings even toward psychiatrists, presuming that the etiquette for interaction stemming from wiser and more knowledgeable fellow-patients has more utility than official standards for the doctor-patient relationship:

> Patients recognize that the best policy is to cooperate with the doctor. Even patients who are hostile to he doctor try to inhibit their feelings. "The patients curse the doctor all day, then act their best when the doctor appears on the ward," observed one patient.[20]

Predictably (and in contrast to the isolation and loneliness of the general hospital), patients in hospitals which produce a collective patient subculture often turn to their colleagues for help and support:

> Troubled by their hallucinations, patients discuss them. They learn that improved patients attribute them to the imagination, but they do not agree. Hence, some hallucinating patients seek help from each other in a common effort to control their "voices."[21]

Sometimes a specific and long-term interest in the client may result in somewhat different patterns of subcultural activity, as for example the patient in a tuberculosis hospital. Here, a relatively long period of time is involved during which the patient perceives that others in the hospital suffer from an identical malady for which there is no immediate release and which calls for great dependency upon the hospital. Patients here are likely to band together—even with significant others "on the outside"—in ways which permit them to live both with their preinstitutional selves and the facts as presented to them by the hospital. Davis describes this process among children stricken with polio:

> A complex of cognitive, situational, and structural influences underlie this shift of perspective . . . the lessening of the child's affective ties with home and his immersion in the hospital's *sub-culture of illness;* and the gradient-like structing of the physiotherapeutic regime, which encouraged child and parents to orient themselves to small-step, progressive gains rather than to the distant goal of recovery (italics ours).[22]

This kind of hospital employs a variety of strategies to ease the patients, as a group, into a collective accommodation consistent with the specific focus and its long-term implications. After describing the many activities which are encouraged on the polio convalescent ward, Davis says:

> The pleasures of sociability after the days of isolation have a telling effect on the children and contribute much to their

positive involvement in the treatment regime. . . . It is against this background of loosened, although by no means severed, affective ties with home that the requisite changes in the child's recovery orientation are brought about.[23]

Thus, the hospital expressing this kind of orientation is ultimately populated by a relatively closely knit and emergent patient cohort which—if the process moves to completion—forms an alliance, however repugnant it may be, with the defining hospital system.

Similar inferences can be drawn from Roth's account of a tuberculosis hospital:

[The patients] often suggest that they are not being moved along as fast as they should. They compare themselves to other patients, they compare the doctor to other doctors, they compare the hospital to other hospitals, all to show that if they were in somebody else's shoes or under somebody else's jurisidiction, they would be farther ahead then the are now. . . .[24]

A slightly different and more poignant expression of this theme is given in Glaser and Strauss' account of a terminal ward in a general hospital. In this setting the accommodative process ends in the most repellant of acceptances: the fact of imminent death. Here the process may begin when the staff communicates to the patient the content of an utterly fictitious future biography—life. In reality, of course, the aim is somehow to get the fatally ill patient to realize and to accept his irreversible fate. Although other patients contribute in an indirect fashion to this realization, they do so via staff members who have taken the experiences of already dead patients and molded them into a model of conduct which the presently dying patients are expected to emulate:

The patient may wish to die in certain ways: without pain, for instance, with dignity, and perhaps in private . . . the staff has its own ideas about the way patients ought to die, involving not merely the physical aspects of dying, but also its moral and stylistic aspects. . . .[25]

These efforts to induce the patient to accept the proper role, as perceived by the hospital, may persist to the very moment of death. Moreover, patient deviations from the prescribed mold—even at the last moment—can be regarded by the staff with disdain. As the authors remark, "the staff appreciates patients who exit with courage and grace,"[26] and by virtue of the hospital's specific and artificially long-term orientation toward the patient, it is usually able to maximize the probability of the dying patient's doing just that.

This strategy of constructing a fictional future biography for physically dying patients is not unlike what occurs at the social psychological level in the total institution so cogently depicted by Goffman. Although the subculture is likely to be of the conflict variety, each patient is more likely to carve out his own ways of "living in the cracks" of the hospital structure through seizing upon techniques of "making out" in the hospital. Although the patient may be present in this kind of hospital for a very long period of time indeed, in a very genuine social psychological sense the patient's life career *is arrested in time.* The patient's future biological life, from the point of view of the staff, is likely to be no different *socially* ten years from now than it was two years ago. By virtue of its definition of the patient's biography, such hospitals come to be populated by living human beings who are dead persons.

It is clear that hospitals bring pressures to bear upon their patients which demand that they conform to some image as to what patients ought to be like and how they should conduct themselves. The imprinting of organizational expectations can hardly be separated from a final matter: the routes that former patients take out of the hospital and how their future life is affected by their experience.

PATIENT BIOGRAPHIES AND POST-HOSPITAL IDENTITIES

As Thomas Scheff has pointed out, hospitals tend to act upon their conceptions of what patients should be like *as if* these conceptions were replicas of reality. In so doing, they define the situation in such a manner that options for the patients are minimized for both their residency in the hospital and their post-hospital existence.

> One of Balint's conclusions is that there is an apostolic function, i.e., that doctors in some ways act as apostles, seeking to proselytize their patients into having the kinds of diseases that the doctors think are conceivable in their cases. . . . If the doctor has the opportunity of seeing [patients] . . . before they settle down to a definite organized illness, he may observe that these patients, so to speak, offer or propose illnesses, and that they have to go on offering new illnesses. . . .[27]

Illness behavior can be much in the nature of a self-full-filling prophecy to the degree that authoritative persons communicate by deed and by gesture how the ill person should act. The doctor *may* operate in terms of a rigid set of expectations, *or* on the basis of a more flexible and negotiative frame of reference. The imprinting of hospital expectations upon patients can hardly be discussed without its logical outcome: the resulting stigmata which remain a part of the patient once he leaves the hospital. Goffman, for example, discussed the role of stigma as it may later affect the person:

> Thus, a one-legged girl, prone to many inquiries by strangers concerning her legs, developed a game called "Ham and Legs" in which the play was to answer an inquiry with a dramatically preposterous explanation. . . . "Questions about how I lost my leg used to annoy me, so I developed a stock answer that kept these people from asking further: I borrowed some money from a loan company and they are holding my leg for security!"[28]

Only through conjecture can we argue that such a specific and long-lasting stigma can best be imprinted in an institution such as the general hospital with a telling and highly specific focus upon the patient, and others in which patients are cast into roles which pre-exist in the mind's eye of the staff even before the patient arrives on the scene. They are specific in their content, limited in scope, and allow for little invention on the part of the patient. Similar processes of patient typification have been observed to take place in the obstetrical hospital—no less specifically focused than is the general hospital:

> the spatial and temporal organization of the service seemed to be geared to cast the incoming patient into a role and mood that would allow the personnel of the service to behave in the ways which they had learned to expect that they should . . . this process was accomplished apparently less by verbal instruction, or even by informal socialization processes, than by the erection of both physical and symbolic barriers to the undesired behaviors and attitudes.[29]

Such processes, of course, find their counterpart in the nice diagnostic distinctions and programmed treatment which accompany them. Not only does this kind of hospital orient toward the patient in a highly specific fashion, but the patient's capacity to function in a variety of other spheres is well regulated. Though the reluctant patient may object to the narrow scope of autonomy permitted him, he may in no significant way take part in forming his own conduct repertory in the hospital.

This does not mean that the patient in the general hospital is *always* compliant. It means only that deviations from the imprinted patient role are effectively countered by the staff in ways which help to insure conformity. One of the more noticeable strategies is to label the defiant patient in ways which shed scorn and indignation upon him, and which arouse guilt and shame in him. The patient who demands too much medication is a "crock"; the one failing to respond to proper treatment is a "malingerer"; the loquacious victim of Korsakov's disease is "disrespectful to the physician"; even the patient who dies too soon, too late, or with too little dignity, is an ingrate.

In spite of all this, the general hospital patient usually carries with him no sociopsychological visible stigma when he returns to normal life. While he may wish to talk about his operation with friends and family, the account usually falls only upon polite ears. The event, from the point of view of the listener, is over and finished, and the patient is patient no longer. He is seen as "repaired" and returned as far as possible to his pre-hospital self.

In more broadly oriented hospitals, however, the expectancies of the staff are less clear, less uniform, and allow for a variety of social types to arise among the patient population. More important, the patient helps to mold his own medical imprint by negotiating with the staff for the creation of new and inventive roles. First, the refracted nature of the hospital's focus upon the patient's life space precludes a specific stigmata. Staff members are likely to approach patients not only with an open mind but also with a modulated authoritative posture. In discussing the diagnostic procedures in one such hospital, the authors say:

> Terms such as free-choice, free-lance, or self-selected programs were generally preferred to convey the idea that the client was free to work out his own destiny and to make use of the accessibility of facilities and personnel as he saw fit. In a like manner, *personnel were also defined as free of any particular responsibility to the client other than the general expectation of being receptive and responsive to him* (italics ours).[30]

It is precisely this absence of predetermined conceptions of what patients ought to be like—except that they shall be active participants in working their own fate—that distinguishes the hospital with an ill-defined interest in the patients' life space. Here, negotiation with the staff is necessary to carve out a role which is not only consistent with the general ideology of total care and the ethic of patient autonomy which prevails but also congruent with the ever present need for order. Although Harry Stack Sullivan declared that the "burden of responsibility lies with the more mature," the burden carried by the least mature can be very great indeed in this kind of hospital.

The question of the accommodation of the patient to his post-hospital life can be most poignant in hospitals which attempt to intervene in their patient's future life for a longer period of time. On the whole, the longer the patient is retained as hospital property—either physically or organizationally—the more he must cope with this problem. Post-hospital stigmata of very special kinds can arise. They often give rise to a rich and varied etiquette for interaction which has to do with the ways the patient must continue to live a dual life—partially as former patient, and partially as a "normal."

We have in mind, for example, what often occurs in the case of the blind, the deaf, alcoholics, drug addicts, and others defined as chronically ill. The stigma resulting from hospitalization is likely to result in *patient colonization* in the post-hospital world, the learning of gestures and mannerisms with which the former client identifies himself to others like him and to "normals," ideas of permanent difference which prohibit full engagement in the social system of which they may once have been a part.

In his discussion of institutions for the blind, Scott remarks:

> Rehabilitators of the blind have the same beliefs about blindness that the layman does [who] are not agents of social change. *They are agents of the community who make blind persons out of people who cannot see.* Their product is a dependent, helpless person who, because of his trained incapacity, requires the sheltered protection of agencies and asylums for the blind (italics ours).[31]

Similar implications of long-term intervention for post-hospital stigmata are implied by Goffman's remarks about the former polio patient:

> Here the medical profession is likely to have the special job of informing the infirm who he is going to have to be. . . . Post-stigma acquaintances may see him simply as a faulted person . . . attached to a conception of what he once was, [and] may be unable to treat him either with formal tact or with familiar full acceptance.[32]

What we wish to convey may be done more easily by exploiting Lemert's classic analysis of deviance: the hospital which attempts to intervene in the patient's future biography may succeed in moving its patients from primary to secondary deviation—from a passing defect in normal functioning to semi-illness as a way of life. This, in turn, necessitates the development of forms of post-hospital organization to tie the members symbiotically to the normal community, and also to the institution which produced their permanent deviance in the first place.

The profound effects that hospital-produced stigmata can have upon the lives of former patients is perhaps no better illustrated than in Edgerton's sensitive study of the mentally retarded ex-patients of Pacific State Hospital:

> [The stigmata] almost inevitably results in reduction of all subsequent interaction to a less complex level than the normal person would otherwise have attempted . . . the normal person who becomes aware of the incompetence of the former patient regularly switches his mode of speech to a condescending tone and a simplified content. The normal person "talks down" and sometimes even attempts a form of "baby talk" as might a colonial Englishman in talking to "native" servants. . . . Interaction is reduced to a plane upon which the normal person asks few questions, utilizes the simplest possible vocabulary, avoids complexities of humor, and assumes that the former patient has almost no knowledge of what is commonplace, much less what is intricate, in the world.[33]

The humiliation of having the character of one's whole future life defined by a long-term experience with an organization such as a hospital can be dealt with in several ways: by the banding-together of former patients into clique-like groups which relive their experience, by developing relationships with benefacting groups in the normal community, and by periodically re-establishing links with the hospital which had such a profound effect upon their lives. Edgerton goes on to illustrate saliently and graphically the stigmatizing result of a period of residency in a hospital with a pointed and long-term orientation toward patients:

> For the ex-patient of an institution for the mentally retarded . . . has been accused and found guilty of being so stupid that he was considered incompetent to manage his own life. As a consequence, he has been confined in an institution for the mentally incompetent. . . . The label of mental retardation not only serves as a humiliating, frustrating, and discrediting stigma in the conduct of one's life in the community, but it also serves to lower one's self-esteem to such a nadir of worthlessness that the life of a person so labelled is scarcely worth living.[34]

Hospitals of all kinds intervene in the lives of their patients in a variety of ways. Some focus specifically on a selected aspect of the patient's social personality, while others are more broadly oriented and attempt to reshape the whole person. Some hospitals attempt only a short-term intervention, while others connect themselves to their patients' future life in most profound ways and for a very long period of time.

As we have attempted to show, each form of intervention the hospital undertakes has far-reaching consequences for the internal structure of hospitals, as well as for the course of hospital life as it unfolds on a day-to-day basis.

Perhaps of more pressing importance, however, is the fact that the nature of a hospital's intervention can have dramatic effects not only upon what the patient shall be as a hospital resident but also upon his fate as a discharged ex-patient. The relationships of a hospital to its external environments (including former patients) are similarly informed by its orientations toward its patients.

The issue of hospitals and their ex-patients—especially as it relates to present efforts to achieve inter-hospital contact and collaboration—is addressed in the following chapter.

8

Orientations toward Clients and Interorganizational Relationships

The answer to the question "Who governs?" . . . is quite literally nobody. The system after a fashion runs. Nobody runs it.

NORTON LONG, *Community Leadership and Decision-Making*

The difficulties encountered in mobilizing community health organizations for collective action are no less than those met in the case of civil rights (which Long was referring to specifically). The almost total absence of effective and continuing collaboration between hospitals is matched only by the paucity of analytical tools by which this situation may be understood, not to mention altered.

In spite of this, medical organizations in American communities are today confronted with potentials for program expansion unparalleled in the history of this country. Federally inspired programs—ranging from community mental health clinics, to grants for the establishment of regional medical complexes—involve operational scope and financial magnitude of monumental proportions. So large are they, indeed, that traditional forms of organization seem in most instances unable to engage these new opportunities and mandates with any present degree of effectiveness. Long may be correct in his contention that any strategy short of direct and centralized authority capable of *commanding* the desired outcome is certain to be second best. Nonetheless, the millennium (or Armageddon, depending on your point of view) of an organization of medical organizations is but vaguely discernible today. For now, the fate of inter-organizational processes and needs is retained, in piecemeal fashion, in the hands of those who run the many separate health institutions in the local community.

Given this simple fact, the obvious sociological challenge has to do with discovering those processes and structures which inhibit or enhance relations between separate health organizations. The more pressing practical matter hinges on the ways and extent to which these inhibiting and enhancing factors can be purposely turned so as to maximize the potentialities which inhere in the elaborate technology of medicine. For as is so frequently pointed out, the immediate problems in the field of health are *organizational* ones.

Of prime importance in mitigating against effective collaboration between hospitals and other medical organizations is the structure of metropolitan communities themselves. High population density seems always to result in increased specialization of function and divisiveness, hardly conducive to planned integration and collaboration. Moreover, the organizations which mushroom in metropolitan communities usually arise in response to the special needs of specially defined segments of the community. With but rare exception, the community health complex, traditionally, has been geared not toward integration and collaboration but rather toward a condition of accommodation which sometimes approaches conflict. In the field of health it is not unusual for hospitals to compete for scarce resources and to lay claims to distinctive clientele as well. Hospitals must also develop and maintain client referral systems, both for reasons of medical economics and to maintain and continue the special place which has been carved out in the total health system of the community. The maintenance of a client referral system results, of course, in the need for hospitals to develop functional relationships with the organization of the medical profession in the community in both its individual and organizational personifications.

The typical community general hospital is not a community institution in any sense of the word. Rather, it is the property of highly specialized and differentiated segments of the population, generally accessible only in moments of crisis to those who are not usually within its orbit.

In contrast to the present situation, which holds at least the promise of relative financial abundance, most hospitals— sometimes out of need—have operated for many years with a depression mentality, anticipating scarcities and countering this expectation with strategies of hoarding both facilities and personnel. This tradition of perceived scarcity leads not only to a series of gentlemen's agreements concerning the allocation of collectivized funds in short supply, mutually understood priorities as to the services which each hospital shall offer, but also to the development of clearly articulated differences among hospitals about the kind of treatment credo which shall inform appeals made to clients, to potential supporters, and to the reservoir of available staff members. Divisive specialization—consistent with high population density as well as with the state of medical technology—is *the* distinctive earmark of the medical system in metropolitan communities.

A dilemma, therefore, lies in the fact that medical institutions in most communities have developed historically against a backdrop of conflict, competition, and divisiveness. But the increasing "nationalization" in the fields of health demands— if not complete consensus and total subjugation of the parochial interests of separate hospitals to a more global conception of need—at least an effective and meaningful accommodation to the requirements of an integrated conception of health services. Indeed, the language of Public Law 89–749 is quite clear in its language and in its implications:

> The Congress declares that fulfillment of our national purpose depends on promoting and assuring the highest level

of health attainable for every person [and] that attainment of this goal depends on an *effective* partnership, involving close inter-governmental collaboration, official and voluntary efforts, and participation of individuals and organizations. . . .[1]

Perhaps of even more telling importance is the stipulation that the agencies charged with developing these overarching medical plans are expected to:

provide for encouraging cooperative efforts among governmental or nongovernmental agencies, organizations and groups concerned with health services, facilities, or manpower, and for cooperative efforts between such agencies, organizations, and groups and similar agencies, organizations, and groups in the fields of education, welfare, and rehabilitation.[2]

Finally, legislation provides that these goals shall be attained:

without interference with existing patterns of private professional practice of medicine, dentistry, and related healing arts.[3]

Partially as a result of constraints such as these, our concern in this chapter with inter-hospital relationships is informed by the proposition that the success of large-scale health programs is contingent upon inter-organizational contact and collaboration.

We shall first examine some aspects of this issue as may be derived from the client biography model. Following that, we shall explore some implications of differential orientations toward patients for maximizing contact, dialogue, and cooperation among the health organizations of a community.

PATIENT BIOGRAPHIES AND HOSPITAL REFERENCE SETS

All organizations, to a greater or lesser extent, take account of *other* organizations in coming to decisions about their clients. No organization makes decisions completely *in vacuo.* On the contrary, all organizational decisions are based partially upon the focal organizations's attempt to include those on the outside—either literally or symbolically. To the extent that a hospital's reference set expands, that is the degree to which it loses effective and exclusive control over its own *internal* system—both process and structure. Further, to the extent that *many* hospitals in the same community expand their spheres of decision making, that can be a crude measure of the emergence of a meaningful inter-hospital system.

Let us propose, now, that the relative *size* of a hospital's reference set is a function of the hospital's orientations toward its patients as shown in Table 13.

TABLE 13

Orientations toward Clients		Size of Reference Set	
Lateral	Longitudinal	Operative	Administrative
—	—	small	small
+	+	large	large
—	+	small	large
+	—	large	small

Again, the specific and short-term focus of the general hospital permits the organization to devise a decision-making system from which other organizations are quite effectively excluded. Its spheres of operational and administrative activities are neatly circumscribed and hardly ever impinge upon other health organizations in the community. Taken in the aggregate, if a community contained hospitals *exclusively* of this type, its medical system would be made up of a "mechanical" division of labor which would operate precisely as the kind of "system nobody runs" alluded to by Norton Long.

Just the reverse would seem to be true in the case of the more broadly and long-term oriented hospital. Here, the wide scope of intervention in the client's life space and the indeterminant span of time for which such intervention is intended requires such a hospital to be super sensitive to other agencies and institutions in the community. This kind of hospital's work—both administrative and operational—impinges upon and overlaps with that of numerous other organizations in the surrounding environment. This means that the "focal" organization quite literally includes other organizations in its decision-making structure. For this reason, at least some of its decisions will derive from its reactions to and perceptions of the definitions and expectations of other institutions. Again, if one were to imagine a community medical system made up only of this type of hospital, it would be an organic system containing overlapping spheres of activities, and a minimal division of labor in which the fate of hospital *A* is quite truly in the hands of hospital *B* and vice versa.

Let us take but one example—patient referral systems—in order to illustrate more concretely what is involved. The typical community general hospital has a patient referral system which can best be described as *deus ex machina.* Patients appear for treatment without any significant effort on the part of the hospital itself. Obviously this occurs because the staff physicians, who are also doctors in private practice, *individually* supply the hospital with patients. Hence, in solving its *staffing* problem, the short-term general hospital quite magically and automatically solves its "input" problem. Its "output" mechanisms are equally simple and nearly automatic. The quick-repair patient is merely discharged, usually into the hands of those family members who accompanied him when he first arrived. In addition, the brief period of time spent in such a hospital does not require that the patient's ties with significant others be either severed upon institutionalization, or repaired and re-established upon impending discharge. As a result of this, the general hospital is in a uniquely fine position to devote nearly all of its energies to perfecting its core-technology without the encumbrances which must occur when both inputs and outputs must be deliberately addressed. More important, however, is the fact that this kind of patient referral and discharge process serves quite effectively to insulate the hospital from contact with other organizations.

Now the more broadly oriented and long-term hospital is likely to contain a quite different set of input and output problems, and especially so in the case of "innovative" hospitals, teaching-research hospitals, and others which—because of their elaborate goals and methods—normally *select* patients on some basis or other. There is the additional contingency that these kinds of hospitals normally contain a combination of full-time medical staffs *and* rotating interneships. What they lack, therefore, is a cadre of practicing medical professionals —each with his own private clientele—to serve as the reservoir of patients. In these cases, input is a problem which must be organizationally met, usually through the elaboration of a unit in the hospital which is responsible for locating suitable patients and routing them to the institution. As a result, the common strategy is for the hospital to reach "out" toward *other organizations* rather than to individuals as is the case with the general hospital staff. Moreover, the long-term intervention which is intended requires that the incoming patient's extra-hospital associations and identities must not only be severed and a new hospital identity established, it means also that the patient must be resocialized, or deinstitutionalized in addition to being made "well." This process of returning the long-term patient to the community implies that the discharge phase is just as problematic as is the intake phase. This, in turn, means that the hospital must establish knowledge of and contact with organizations and agents at "both ends" of the treatment process. One final point to make in regard to this example: It is obvious that many such hospitals, in solving *its own input problem,* either by plan or by accident solves another organization's output problem. And the corollary: In solving its output problem it must necessarily resolve *another* organization's input problem. This fact then sets the stage for the development of symbiotic relationships between groups of hospitals and for the shifting of goals and policies of the individual members of the set.

To return to our more general discussion: A further consequence of differences in the size of reference sets is found in the degree to which extra-organizational feedback is an essential feature of the hospital. The long-term hospital, for example, though it attempts to achieve a continuing and perhaps even permanent imprint upon the patient, is seldom able to maintain full and effective control over the fate of its lost clients. Upon their physical departure from the hospital they become the property of other organizations and institutions. Some of these may not be medical institutions. In its efforts to assess the worth of its work upon the patient, this kind of hospital must rely upon feedback from other institutions. Hence, the long-term hospital may use such information not only as a means of maintaining contact with its former patients but also as a way of evaluating its own effectiveness and perhaps changing itself internally on the strength of what a separate and different organization says about it. Implications of such a pattern can be equally manifold for inter-hospital collaboration as well as for traditional conceptions of single hospital autonomy and independence.

In sum, differences in orientation toward patients' lives—both present and future—result in different-size reference sets for decision making and, ultimately, to quite different reliance upon extra-hospital feedback. This, in turn, can dramatically alter the hospitals.

It would serve no useful purpose here to continue an elaboration of the external linkages of hospitals at this level of abstraction. Partially because of the current efforts to ameliorate the health problems of large segments of the population, there is more justification in raising a series of questions more concretely related to the capabilities of hospitals for effective and meaningful inter-organizational collaboration. Though it is true that medical organizations tend to function in isolation, the fact is that national programs in health and welfare demand collaborative arrangements. It is useful to make the distinction between collaboration at the policy-administrative and at the operating-implementing level. While both may be desirable and perhaps essential, they do not necessarily take place together. For example, separate hospitals may indeed engage in collaborative efforts on general fiscal matters, channeling of information concerning plans for long-range development, and other administrative matters which serve essentially to insure, in a relative sense, the maintenance of the status quo. But they may not collaborate at all at the operational level (at the point of direct contact with the patient) through joint utilization of scarce professional personnel, or by the sharing of newly acquired treatment knowledge, and the like. The reverse may occur, though it is likely that administrative collaboration has more often taken place than has joint operational participation.

It is of further use to make the distinction between formal and informal inter-hospital collaboration. By formal we mean those processes by which members of two or more organizations engage in relationships with one another *in their capacities as members of their hospitals*. By informal is meant those strategies of inter-hospital contact in which the collaborators act in some capacity *other than as organizational members*. Hence, it is the substance of the interaction between hospitals not its structural form which forms the distinction.

Let us argue that these modes of inter-hospital collaboration are closely related to the nature of the organizations' interests in the patient's life, present and future. We suggest specifically that the four types of hospital differ in their propensities for different kinds of collaboration as shown in Table 14.

TABLE 14

Orientations toward Clients		*Modes of Collaboration*			
		Formal		Informal	
Lateral	Longitudinal	Operating	Admin.	Operating	Admin.
—	—	no	no	yes	yes
+	+	yes	yes	no	no
—	+	yes	no	no	yes
+	—	no	yes	yes	no

The specific and short-term focused institution— the community general hospital for example—typically has little propensity for formal and direct collaboration with other hospitals at *either* the administrative or the operative levels. The specificity of its interest in the patient and its concern with finely discriminated strategies of care—sometimes constituting a cost gradient as well—tend to make such hospitals isolated professional islands in the community. They may, however, be thrust into dialogue with one another through intermediary organizations such as the local medical society or the local hospital planning councils. Nonetheless, the interstitial character of such bridging organizations makes them fertile grounds for the introduction of themes in inter-hospital dialogue not directly addressed to patient care per se. These can range from ethnic and racial differences to the firmly encrusted barriers between public and private sponsorship, to even more subtle manifestations of local community power cliques and spheres of influence. Perhaps even more important, it is in the highly focused acute hospital that a major avenue of operational collaboration is *least* likely to occur, i.e., the joint appointment of medical personnel to two or more medical establishments. Indeed, the competitive character of the typical general hospital mitigates against utilizing this promising mode of strategies to follow their departed clients. "Checking" on patients requires the development of administrative mechanisms for getting information from other organizations which may later be responsible for the welfare of the patient.

Partially as a result of such forces, the short-term acute general hospital normally stands as a splendid pillar of isolation in the community with little interest or even capacity to develop master plans for health care with other organizations.[4]

All of this is true only at the *formal* level. Hospitals such as these are usually caught up in a complex network of informal relationships which may include the local medical society and health insurance programs in the community, the major institutional establishments via the members of its Board of Trustees, as well as whatever local community power structures as do exist. We do not mean to imply that the specifically focused and short-term hospital does not engage in contact or dialogue with *other* hospitals; we mean merely that *control* over the kind and extent of collaborative activities has been given over to *extra* hospital persons and agencies.

The more broadly oriented and long-term hospital stands as the most contrasting type. The elite psychiatric hospital, for example, is customarily involved in a massive and sometimes conflicting set of operative and administrative links establishing *rapprochement* between hospitals.

The consequences for the patient of this high degree of specialization can be manifold. Robb, for example, has described just this pattern of inter-agency specialization as it affects the care and treatment of children:

> If one looks at the consequence of this on problems which overlap or fall between two functional areas, one often gets an impression of a very low level of efficiency; like an imperfectly adjusted lathe which cuts out only part of the total pattern. It is all rather too reminiscent of the famous hospital bulletin, "The operation was completely successful, but, unfortunately, the patient died."[5]

The functionally specific pattern of medical services may

result in the efficient organization of the separate and isolated hospitals in the community, each considered separately. But such a pattern can hardly be expected to result in efficiency at the total community level. The reverse may in fact be true: The very efficiency of separate institutions with their loyalties to special segments of the population may result in duplication of expensive services, and thus be detrimental to the needs of the community which they attempt to serve independently of one another.

Because such hospitals do have a short-term interest in their patients, they need not devise linkages at *both* the formal and informal levels. The wide range of professional personnel it contains tends to extend professional contacts into other similarly oriented hospitals. Indeed, communities which contain several such hospitals—all attempting to intervene in the patient's present and future life—are likely to have a pool of professional persons whose skills are drawn upon by a large number of separate organizations. A long-term interest in the client's future biography also means that such a hospital has to devise ways of establishing working relationships with other organizations which may ultimately be held responsible for the later career of the patient.[6]

A specifically oriented short-term hospital is likely to have few established linkages with family welfare agencies, nursing homes, the juvenile court, and the like, while persons working in hospitals attempting a broader and longer-term intervention in the life space of their patients are often intimately tied in with many other institutions. For example, a study of patient orientations in psychiatric hospitals found that:

> Extension of services to the clients of *other* organizations was associated with (1) recent organizational establishment, (2) large professional staffs, and (3) small administrative components. In terms of the perspective examined here, plus-lateral and minus-longitudinal hospitals included the clients of *other* organizations while the minus-lateral and plus-

longitudinal hospitals limited their focus *(operational)* on their own patients.[7]

To depict the situation somewhat differently, this kind of hospital might be characterized as centrifugal at both the operative and administrative levels. That is, the elegance and complexity of its orientation toward the spatial and temporal aspects of the patient's life is matched by an equally complex and elaborate set of external structural extensions. And just as its internal system is fraught with conflict and dissension, so too its external arrangements are likely to be highly unstable and changeable. Of special note in this regard, stemming from the coincidence of *both* broad and long-term interests, is that such external conflicts of hospitals are likely to include confrontations and clashes *between* the operative and administrative ethics as they struggle for priority in the external environment. This is in contrast to the more clearly delineated external relationships of the typical short-term general hospital, more likely to be marked by consensus achieved through the mediating structures of the larger community. There appear to be variable relations between a hospital's structural extensions in "time" and "space" toward other organizations and its functional commitments to its patients.

PATIENT BIOGRAPHIES AND INTERORGANIZATIONAL CONTACTS

We would expect that a similarity of orientation toward patients by two different hospitals would be likely to enhance collaborative activities, while the coming together of two or more contrasting types of hospitals would inhibit collaboration, or perhaps even lead to open hostility and conflict.

In the field of rehabilitation, for example, illustrations may be found of these divergent types. Deliberately contrived programs of collaboration involving the consolidation of different rehabilitation agencies—such as organizations for the blind, the mentally retarded, or the physically handicapped—often founder at the operational level. This ineffective outcome may be explained by the fact that rehabilitation agencies are differentially committed to the life space of their clients—some manifesting a broad interest and some a narrowly constricted one. This implies wide differences among such agencies in both their internal structural characteristics and their prevailing patterns of interactions, especially as related to the operational sphere. What appears to account for the collaborative effort in the first place is a common interest in the future career of the client. One logical outcome of this duality is harmony and effective dialogue at the administrative level, but a great deal of conflict and dissension at the operational level. Furthermore, over time this condition may become characterized by elaborate administrative superstructures rather than by increased operational effectiveness.

An additionally clear example of this process is discernible in the recent history of the National Mental Health Association. Until a short time ago, it existed only as loosely associated congeries of autonomous local mental health societies. Some of the patron groups were broadly and others narrowly committed to their clientele. They shared, however, a common long-term interest in the careers of their locally defined client groups. The original move toward officially established cooperation came through the New York office and has persisted most notably at the administration, communication, and fund-raising level. So far, indeed, has the "nationalization" of the movement gone that most of the originally autonomous local societies provide little or no service to clients. We hasten to add, however, that this administrative system does ultimately result in the delivery of service to clients, but mainly in indirect forms by way of research activities supported through the association's fund-raising, public mental health education programs, and so forth.

On the whole, the local societies function at the present

time merely as linkages in a nationwide administrative system. It is important to note that this decline of direct service function and the pre-eminence of administrative activities have resulted in a dramatic shift in the sources of personnel recruitment and the staffing patterns of the once service-providing local societies.

These remarks about inter-organizational collaboration are designed to suggest some of the logical outcomes for collaboration problems likely to arise when organizations with different commitments to the client biography impinge upon each other's spheres of activity.

Considerations such as these—inexhaustive and highly speculative as they must be—seem to lead to a major implication from which a number of important consequences arise: Hospitals have different capacities for effective and meaningful collaboration at both the operational and administrative levels. These capacities derive ultimately from the ways and extent to which the hospital chooses to intervene in the life of the patient. Such an assertion is of little practical utility except as it is viewed from the understanding that present large-scale programs in health and welfare make few if any such distinctions. However, effective collaboration is asked for, if not demanded, from all, or nearly all, of the generic organizations in the medical complex. Though it may be too early to comment on the recent health and welfare programs, it seems clearly the case that in too many instances the older tradition of inter-agency conflict or purely administrative pre-eminence has to a marked degree undermined many such programs and added further foment to our troubled metropolitan communities.

We cannot pretend that the client biography perspective set forth holds the solution to the problems of how to achieve effective and meaningful inter-organizational collaboration. It is suggested only that as a sensitizing concept it contributes to a more integrated understanding that issues of hospital autonomy and interaction are closely related to both the structural characteristics of organizations and the interaction of patients with hospital representatives.

THE CONCEPT OF "COMMAND" AND INTER-AGENCY COLLABORATION

One alternative—pointed to by Norton Long in the field of civil rights—is to *command* compliance to plans for optimal medical care delivery through authoritative reorganization of the body politic in metropolitan communities. As logically sound as such a solution may be, forces too numerous to list here presently mitigate against a full realization of the obvious potentials, at least in the foreseeable future.

However, attempts to "metropolitanize" separate spheres of public health activities in large cities represent faltering but nonetheless forward steps in this direction. These are often piecemeal in nature, involving first the centralization of administrative functions in the core city and then the exercise of central authority over discretely defined health related phenomena. It is (parenthetically and in our terminology) a drift toward a codification of the minus-lateral/plus-longitudinal orientation. Though such incorporations may in fact result in more uniform, and perhaps more efficient, standards and criteria as regards sanitation, inoculation, and so on, public health spheres as presently defined do not directly touch the main problems of health care and medical organizations. First, public health departments, almost by definition, do not directly serve clients in the same way that practicing physicians and hospitals do. Rather, they are in the service of the "public welfare" and the fact that they must occasionally confront *persons* is really quite incidental to their primary mission. This is obviously not true for those departments of health charged with the care of institutionalized mental patients. But here again the *primary* charge is more the public welfare than the treatment of patients. Second, public health departments—whether centralized or not and with the exception just noted—simply do not have the masonry and equipment which is critical as a physical place for the coming together of hospital and patient.

As more diseases of the chronic type are drawn into the orbit of public concern, it seems likely that public health departments and units *will* become directly involved in the treatment of patients (as for example in the use of artificial kidney machines), in addition to their traditional role as overseers of the state of public sanitation. As direct treatment of clients by public health officials increases, so too will the public ownership of physical facilities as a locus for the coming together of clients and the medical representatives of the body politic. For the moment, however, the exercise of command in the field of health is highly scattered and only occasionally focused upon specific health problems and disease entities.

SELECTED ORGANIZATIONS AND INTER-AGENCY COLLABORATION

A second alternative—and one for which there is considerable precedent—is to assess the structural characteristics of specific health organizations in terms of the potentials they may hold for affecting meaningful collaboration. In this sense, reference is made once again to the client biography perspective insofar as its consequences may enhance inter-agency collaboration. Deliberate selection of hospitals on the basis of commonalities of orientations toward the spatial or temporal aspects of the patient's biographical career can well be expected to increase collaboration at either the operational or administrative levels, or both. The notion of selecting potentially collaborative organizations on the basis of these particular structural dimensions, or any number of others, is a dramatic departure from what has recently occurred in the health agency field.

In recent efforts to achieve organizational integration at the regional level, the idea of judiciously selecting appropriately prepared organizations has been renounced in favor of what can be termed "blanket plans" for organizational integration. That is, all or nearly all health institutions in an area—regardless of any realistic assessment of their collaborative potentials—have been the target of such programs. This may, in part, account for not only the strife and conflict which often mark the birth of such regional programs, but also their usually brief life span and the finality of their death. Without the exercise of political command, it may be utterly visionary to expect all health agencies in a county, state, or regional area to have the same interest in, capacity for, or tolerance with such plans. Reference is made here to the Kalaska County, Michigan, and the Hunterdon, New Jersey, experiments, among others.[8] The logic of the client biography conception and the reflections of Levine and White, Thompson and McEwen, and others reveal that instances of direct conflict with and open opposition to such massive plans are to be expected.

It does seem reasonable that effective selection of potentially collaborating hospitals might begin by taking the organization's existing commitment to their clientele as a point of departure. An organization's capacity to extend itself to the point of official contact and inter-action with other organizations is related to the interactional dynamics which characterize the participation of its patient groups in the hospital structure. Such a capacity is also more or less limited by the characteristics of both its operational and administrative lines and the many structural features related to them. All appear to arise out of the organization's original orientation to its clients. And because health organizations, even general hospitals, *do* differ in their orientation to clients, it may be Pollyanna folly to impose a blanket plan for collaboration over the multi-organizational complex. Such a strategy invites conflict and defeat.

Indeed, a specific focus upon the patient, and especially the selection of client characteristics judged to be appropriate to the domain of the hospital, can be useful in drawing together disparate agencies and institutions in a workable and persisting system of collaboration and comprehensive care. For example, the Kaiser Foundation medical care system *for its employees* appears to have drawn into its orbit both hospitals and services which probably would not have been possible under the blanket-plan concept.[9] The same is probably true of the Ford Hospital in Detroit. The New York HIP and the Family Health Maintenance program of the Montefiore Hospital and Medical Center is yet another example of the potential integrating power of a focus upon client characteristics.[10] Finally, the mushrooming preventive health and group practices occurring throughout the country appear to be providing highly comprehensive and long-term preventive medical care. They share the common aspect of selecting clients on the basis of considered criteria—low risk not necessarily being one of them. If, for example, one equates what we have here called plus-laterality with comprehensive care, it is important to note that comprehensive care programs appear to have arisen and been effectively sustained in instances when the institutions involved have focused specifically upon some client characteristic—age, ethnicity, work status. By holding constant, "controlling for," if you will, some significant dimensions of the patient population, the hospital is able to address more of the total patient. It is precisely this focus upon the client which seems likely to enhance the probability of comprehensive care, a broad orientation toward the patient's life, developing across discrete organizational boundaries.

TAILORING PROGRAMS TO HOSPITAL CHARACTERISTICS

Yet a third alternative method of extending and expanding medical services through collaborative efforts between separate institutions is to bring the forces engendering changes in line with the potentialities which already exist in the present medical system. Rather than imposing massive "blanket programs" without regard to the special problems of individual hospitals, facilities and resources for expanded care might be made available, while the specific uses can be determined partially by the participating institutions and agencies themselves.

There are two recent and dramatic, though quite different, ways in which this strategy has been applied. The first, only indirectly related to the field of health, are the several programs subsumed under the Office of Economic Opportunity. The second is Medicare.

In the first instance, only the most general objectives and goals were delineated. The specific content and procedures toward their attainment were left largely in the hands of the organizational complex in the cities. In fact, in many programs the operating funds are withheld by statute until the community institutions *together* present a viable and workable plan consistent with the broad outline of the federal program. In the light of the traditional divisiveness between separate institutions in communities, their characteristically competitive relationships, and their variant definitions of and orientations toward clients, it is not at all surprising that coordinate plans have seldom been forthcoming. Funds have not been allocated, clients are denied access to important services, communities lose a significant amount of service-supporting resources, ambitious programs remain unimplemented, and the separate organizations retain their essentially competitive relationships with one another. This is made even more poignant by the recognition of the losses suffered by all, losses which each attributes to the other's intransigent position with respect to client responsibilities and program aims.

Medicare represents a variant of this process. Here the implementing program was not legitimized *until* such time as it conformed in many respects to the demands made by the institutions, agencies, and professional groups (patients excepted) most directly affected by the innovation. Thus, nursing homes and associations, individual hospitals and hospital associations, the American Medical Association and numerous local medical societies constituted a pluralistic pattern of pressure groups whose activities defined the content of the law as it was finally passed: the now frequent charge that the program is riddled with procedural details (some not entirely free of internal inconsistency and conflict); options as to procedures, content, and funding; alternatives as to length of care provided under alternate conditions and with sliding benefits; that the individual organizations most directly effected can, in very large part, qualify for financial support under the program while implementing it in ways more or less consistent with both their original position of isolation and their chosen orientation toward patients in general.

In spite of deficiencies in both cases—OEO and Medicare— these programs are needed, are of considerable benefit to clients, and are otherwise desirable and worthwhile. We wish only to emphasize some of the unanticipated consequences which arise in the perplexing arena of inter-organizational contact and collaboration. The negotiative strategy of trying to bring federally imposed expectations and opportunities in line with the prevailing system of inter-organizational patterns in health and welfare is to court serious program dilution at best and lack of program implementation at worst.[11]

Before turning to a final consideration of viewing the client as an integrating strategy, let us consider one final alternative in the field of inter-organizational collaboration.

ORGANIZATIONAL INTEGRATION AND THE "BROKER" ROLE

One tactically expedient option is to accept the fact of organizational isolation, program specialization, separate spheres of activity and operational domains. This does not preclude a realization on the part of the separate organizations that new needs do exist for broad based and long-term delivery or service. In fact, the election of a longitudinal orientation toward clients on the part of multiple medical and welfare institutions in a community forces attention to the fact that clientele overlap one another. The same clients appear again and again for different and specialized services in many different settings. These organizations may be structurally unable to alter either their posture toward the client or their relationships with other involved organizations. One way to fill the lacunae is through the use of specially contrived intermediary or "broker" roles which span organizational boundaries.

The field of rehabilitation offers an example of this strategy in the form of the "rehabilitation counselor."[12] The dilemma of the broker role of the rehabilitation counselor, and to some extent of the newly envisaged programs of extended care generally, is that an acceptable organizational model is not yet available. Wesson has commented, "There is not yet an organizational pattern for rehabilitation which is typical of human activity in the sense that the school typifies education or the hospital the practice of medicine."[13] While there is a movement toward the creation of rehabilitation centers, the counselor (who is really the implementer of the new concept of care) must usually function in the context of organizations designed primarily for purposes other than those specifically relevant to rehabilitation. Thus, counselors—and other individual personifications of medical care innovations—are found in schools, hospitals, prisons, employment agencies, and departments of welfare. In the case of rehabilitation, innovative activities are often viewed as viable components of a multi-tude of organizational types and styles. In spite of this funda-mental acceptance, rehabilitation counselors find themselves in organizations geared to other primary purposes. By virtue of the diffuse character of the counselor's orientation to the client the counselor must continually relate to *other* organiza-tional entities. These organizations may be formally structured to service clients or patients in terms of perceptions and atti-tudes not always in accord with the more general objectives and philosophy of the rehabilitation expert.

The development of the rehabilitation center may be viewed as an effort to free the rehabilitation counselor from his basic-ally hostile organizational housing and to provide him an in-stitutional anchorage of sufficient bite that rehabilitation (or other innovative experiments in health and welfare) may have an equal chance to compete in the organizational complex with respect to both resource acquisition and client recruit-ment and conversion. The obvious trap is that in the very process of achieving an organizational home and a lever on the total organizational system, the rehabilitation center may well revert to the very program specialization, clientele mo-nopolies, and interorganizational conflict and diviseness which originally drove the counselor out of the schools, hospitals, and the welfare agencies.

A solution, of course, is to free the counselor—or the individ-ual emissaries of all innovative forms—from *any* identifiable organizational anchorage. That is, to create a genuine broker or intermediary role to make it possible for the new orientation toward clients to be sustained through protecting it from the inroads that are inherently made by full participating mem-bership in an organization. Hence, the broker carries the potential of achieving broader based and longer-term care for patients through mobilizing and integrating the many special services and capabilities of existing isolated— and even antagonistic—organizations. Paradoxically, inter-organizational collaboration may be possible in some instances without re-course to the customary strategies of consolidation, co-opta-tion, merger, or program integration, all of which appear to assume prior conditions of lack of conflict and antagonism.

Perhaps the major pitfall of the broker strategy lies in the fact that the broker—though his commitment is presumably to a declared posture *vis-à-vis* clients—can hardly be expected to spend much of his time directly with clients. He is likely to become basically an administrator, trailing client groups from institution to institution. The broker's peripatetic role isolates him from clients and forces him into continual dia-logue with administrative issues of the organizations to which he is periodically attached. Though there is little evidence which bears directly on this issue, it would seem that the medical care broker is a prime candidate for administrative co-optation and operational goal displacement because of his very isolation from those his mission demands that he ad-dress—the clients.

Paradoxically, however, a successful use of the broker travel-ing between specialized institutions stands a reasonable chance of achieving operational comprehensive care (a broad lateral orientation) while sustaining the fundamentally specific ori-entation of the organizations viewed individually.

FOCUS ON THE PATIENT AS "CLIENT" OR "CUSTOMER"

A deliberate focus on the client in an effort to achieve comprehensive and long-term care involves an exceedingly important change in the customary relationships between the medical system and patients. Specifically, we have in mind the distinction between the patient as "client," on the one hand, and as "customer" on the other. Necessarily, the way the patient is defined has far-reaching consequences for the organization of the medical system and accepted standards of professional conduct.

When the patient is defined as client, he logically must seek out medical care on his own. An implicit and correlate assumption is that the patient can effectively conduct a self-diagnosis and enter rationally into the suitable referral system which then will route him to the proper care-giving practitioner or organization. A functional correlate, of course, is the medical ethic which prescribes that neither the physician nor the hospital may actively *seek out* those persons for whom the potential services are regarded as especially suitable and proper. The exception once again is in the sphere of public health, which is the most contrasting type in terms of mandate to "reach out" and even coerce where necessary. In general, though, the restrictions against the medical doctor's—and all other professionals'—right to "advertise" his wares has its organizational equivalent in the reluctance of hospitals to reach out into the population and differentially select their patients. The prevailing, though now weakened, concept has been that *all* physicians and therefore *all* hospitals are pretty much equivalent, and that *all* clients bear characteristics of equivalent saliency to all medical institutions. The implication is that clients need not choose invidiously or otherwise between doctors and services, and that medical organizations need not select judiciously among the great reservoir of potential clients. Such a perspective assumes also that the referral system by which patients are routed to institutions is efficient in its function. Once this assumption is made, it compels the conclusion that there is nothing amiss in the delivery system of medicine. Hence, efforts to impose blanket integration plans —to integrate indiscriminately *all* medical facilities in a city, a region, or an area—are consistent with the traditional tenets of professional conduct and with the underlying conception of the patient as client.

A critical and perhaps the only point at which the inadequacies of such a conception (and through which its implications for medical organization) can be empirically observed is at delivery of service. For as Scott and Volkart have recently asserted, "To the extent that there is today a 'crisis in American medicine,' as many of our leading periodicals are fond of asserting from time to time, it is not a crisis centering around the quality of medical services as such, but concerns chiefly the organization and distribution of those services."[14] This deficiency can be in large part attributed to the present organizational arrangements in medicine, especially in relation to the existing referral systems.

In any event, the breakdown of the conception of the patient as client must certainly be traced to a beginning with the increased specialization of technology in medicine. The discrete announcements ethically allowed to be printed in newspapers that "Dr. So-and-So Announces the Opening of Practice—Limited to Neurosurgery" is a public admission of the need for client selectivity, as well as an implicit acceptance that the patient is really not in a position to select a practitioner or a hospital wisely or well. However, the fact that the ill person must still turn to his general practitioner in the initial referral process testifies that there have as yet been only modest steps away from the conception of the patient as a prudently selecting client. In our view, the specifically focused and short-term institution—the typical general hospital for example—epitomizes the organizational embodiment of the patient seen as client. Hospitals which orient toward the patient's biographical career in different ways represent modifications of this classic view.

The conception of the patient as "customer," however, implies a different set of relationships between the medical system and the populations served. It assumes, first of all, that the patient is in no position to select among unequal and different alternatives in medical care. Second, it assumes that all medical facilities are not equally appropriate for all members of the population. Out of these two assumptions springs the compelling conclusion that different constituent elements in the medical complex must seek ways to *define* their relevant publics and to make their relevance publicly known. Hence, organizations which view patients as customers must reach out to the population—to capture segments of it is perhaps too strong a term—in order to deliver the chosen medical service to the appropriate people. As a result, medical agencies and organizations must extend themselves beyond their traditional organizational boundaries and actively engage in selecting, educating, and ultimately *controlling* their chosen patient-customers. (Patient control is a matter of considerable importance and will be returned to at the close of this book.)

The newly emerging conception of the patient as customer means also that hospitals incorporating such a view must logically denounce a commitment to the classic "magical hand" referral system which had the effect of distributing segments of the population relatively rigidly among the several hospitals in a community, in a pattern that resembled congeries of private "clientele" and went far to mitigate against meaningful inter-organizational dialogue. It is not at all surprising that those organizations and their medical personnel who presently embrace the newer conception of the patient as a customer (requiring guidance and direction in his use of medical service) often represent the elements of the local medical system which stand somehow apart from the traditional medical establishment in a community. One unexplored clue to the possible enhancement of inter-agency collaboration in the health field is precisely this newer conception of the patient as a customer, especially when the customers are those of the population who have but loose ties with the extant referral system or are in those communities with an uncodified local medical power structure or one in the interim period of internal change. Again, such assertions are mere speculation, but the possible consequences stem directly from an altered conception of the patient. We would also suspect that hospitals deviating from the traditional general hospital pattern are probably most susceptible to the internal and external changes which would lead to a view of the patient as a customer rather than as a client.

HOSPITAL CHANGE AND THE ETHICAL PROBLEM OF PATIENT CONTROL

It is hardly possible to predict what predominant organization form is likely to emerge to supplant the traditional highly focused and short-term hospital. To the extent that one does predict, however, there will be profound changes in the prevailing conception of the patient as a client and considerable pressures exerted upon the existing "informal organization of medicine" at the community level. Dissatisfaction with the prevailing patient referral system and greater numbers of experiments in comprehensive care involving interagency collaboration are likely to appear.

It might be fair to predict at this point that whatever alterations might occur along the contemporary life-space axis of our scheme as far as hospitals are concerned, a more elongated time orientation toward patients is a real probability. This is so not only because of the changing age shape of the population and the nature of chronic diseases which call for long-term care, but also because of the numerous pressures toward the expansion of public health responsibilities and the ethic of humanism which increasingly demands effective care in *both* the long and the short-run.[15]

In sum, hospitals, whether they attempt to address the total patient or merely some specifically selected aspect of him, are likely to attempt to maintain their domain over a longer period of time. Our final argument, then, is that a drift from a short toward a long-term orientation carries with it profound ethical implications which cannot be ignored.

As was pointed out earlier, the medical system has both technical and humanistic themes in its traditional underpinning. And the drift toward a broad and comprehensive orientation appears to have very close ideological linkages with the demand for less depersonalized and more humane concern for the total person. The paradox, of course, is that hospitals which attempt to intervene broadly in the patient's life must devise a wide range of control strategies over patients in order to maintain their compliance with regard to as many of those aspects of the patient's contemporary life space which the hospital chooses to address.[16] That is, as the organization's lateral span of interest increases, that is the degree to which the patient becomes subject to potentially coercive control— even though it may be ideologically phrased as being in "his best interests." This loss of patient autonomy in the typical broad based but short-term hospital is finally terminated once the patient departs the institution; his freedom is to some degree lost, but only for a specified period of time.

The long-term hospital has similar implications for the exercise of coercion, but of a quite different order because of the period of time over which the threat of its use persists. The drift toward extended longitudinal intervention in the client's life also has ideological components. But the commitment on the part of a hospital to intervene in the client's life space in the long run carries with it precisely the same need to control the client as characterizes the "laterally" oriented hospital. It is, however, a shared coercion to the extent that more and more long-term service organizations lay claims to the same patient groups, with the patient subject to the controlling efforts of a large number of disparate organizations in which *he may no longer regard himself as holding membership* and whose legitimacy *may be called into question* by him. Now where this occurs in the *public* sphere, the inter-organizational conspiracy of elongated control and coercion may take the form of statutory right to control. At the same time, the public sphere normally includes prescribed mechanisms by which the client may legitimately counter organizational controls, or at least state an appeal exempting him from such control and terminating the organization's grasp upon him.

Where it occurs in the *private* sphere, the exercise of long-term control and coercion more likely takes the form of a conspiracy of persuasion which hardly permits the client to exempt himself effectively. One might suspect, therefore, that one outcome of increased longitudinality of care—when it occurs in the context of a formally contrived organization—may ultimately come to be directed toward those *least likely to resist* effectively: the uninformed, the acquiesent, and other "powerless" segments of the population who see as their only options living with organizational controls, and "colonizing" only to the extent of carving out some modicum of personal autonomy in the interstitial areas of life space to which some organization has not as yet laid a claim. Some of the experiences in the poverty program point out just some of these contingencies under which coercive strategies of control follow on the heels of the best of intentions. For example, in discussing the implications of the all-out effort against mental illness among the poor, Warren Haggstrom cogently argues that the fundamental source of poor peoples' disadvantages in health and *rapprochement* with health institutions is lack of power—an inability to mobilize collectively, an inability to "define the situation," and an inability to erect counter controls and barriers to inhibit violations of privacy and personal autonomy.[17] For if there is an identifiable integrating theme in these new and intense treatment approaches for the poor, it is that agencies can best attack problems of mental illness among the poverty-stricken by exploiting the fact of their powerlessness. The psychiatric worker can approach lower-class potential patients in their homes, the poolroom, the local tavern, or their places of work; and they can be enticed into the agency's orbit without being informed as to what is happening to them. Whether this is likely to become a pattern in medicine remains a moot but important question.

In any case, whatever the orientation of a health institution toward its patients may be and whatever the structural characteristics to which it leads, the organization must still perform system maintenance functions. The long-term institution —partially because of its external linkages with other organizations, and partially because of its public visibility—has a special need in this regard. As Sjoberg says, "The controls exerted by the bureaucrats over members of the lower class are intensified because the office holders are constantly called upon to normalize and stabilize the system with an eye to maintaining the proper public image."[18]

The adoption of a long-term orientation toward the patient's biographical career seems likely to enhance the potentials for interagency contact and collaboration. It may lead also to a more efficient utilization and comprehensive distribution of available medical resources to a wider population base. As a result, health organizations may in fact be freed from their traditional and inhibiting patterns of isolation and competition.

The consumer (the patient) however, may be in danger of being engulfed by a bondage brought about by an awesome organizational revolution.

EPILOGUE

The Role of the
Federal Government

There is little doubt that the federal government is keenly aware of the care and caution with which any kind of massive planning in the field of health must be handled. At the time of writing, it is nearly nine years since the American Public Health Association and the National Health Council began the work which led to the creation of the National Commission on Community Health. These planning functions are just now beginning to take hold in local communities. The six task forces of the National Commission studied and reported on a broad range of health issues, needs, and resources including comprehensive care and the reorganization of medical facilities.[1] Action was clearly intended and action has now begun: The federal government is now in the health pool with both feet, but still in shallow water.

Specific to regionalization, for example, the Guidelines for Regional Medical Programs states, "This is a new program in an exploratory phase. It is expected that policies and procedures will evolve with time. . . . The Division encourages diversity and innovation . . . these purposes should be accomplished without interfering with the patterns of professional practice or hospital administration."[2] As in the original comprehensive health planning legislation of 1966, the need for negotiated accommodation between the old and new forms of medical care delivery is clear.

Again with reference to regionalization, by January 1967, 34 planning grants had been made; 14 more were under review, and by mid-February 4 operational grants had been made. Taken together, the 48 regions included in these programs and grants encompass an estimated 90 per cent of the American geography, and perhaps even more of the available medical technology.

The legislation stipulates that funds are for research, facilities, and "demonstration" activity, with the implication that the "patient" will be only marginally involved. But the term "demonstration" is open to broad interpretation. Dr. Sidney Farber, for example, remarked that "no one is taking the patient away from his physician . . . [however] we are also interested in all those people who do not have a family physician."[3]

A central idea of the demonstration concept is that successful programs funded by federal money are to be taken over by other agencies in the community. Thus, one result of the demonstration strategy is that *both* patients and existing medical organizations have become sharply vulnerable to change.

The government enters the health field through yet another avenue—the neighborhood health center as developed out of the Office of Economic Opportunity. Structurally, this is at the opposite end of the continuum from the Regional Medical idea. That is, the organization of regions of care is perhaps the most encompassing and "cosmopolitan" new conception yet to appear in the health field, while the neighborhood health center seems to be more patient-oriented and locally focused.

In spite of efforts at both the bottom and the top—neighborhood, local, and comprehensive; regional, cosmopolitan, and more specifically oriented—the findings of one study indicate that only the surface of need is being scratched.[4] Large gaps were found in all medical services. Patients saw the principal need as "a health care facility . . . community oriented" with a "reach-out" program to encourage use of the available services. As is well known, the underprivileged and those otherwise marginal to the mainstreams of society have little such capacity. They seem to need individualized help in using health facilities, a rare feature indeed of existing medical organizations.

In spite of unmet needs and pesky problems such as these, the Poverty Program does seem to be encouraging innovation and locally relevant forms, and there is some probability that this will help stimulate much that is creative and original. It seems important also to point out that most of these newer forms of medical organization, from regionalization down to the neighborhood health center, all demand some degree of collaboration between the public and private sectors of medicine. It may be too early to predict whether the outcomes of joint public and private efforts in the field of health will justify its use as a general mode of financing and reorganization in the future. If it can be shown to work well, it may yield guidelines as how best to capitalize on the advantages of each sector of medicine, while curbing the potentially pernicious effects inherent in complete control by either one or the other.

All the varied and complex grievances about existing medical services hinge in one way or another on that contemporary central dilemma with which this book began, namely, how to achieve a working accommodation of technological sophistication and functional differentiation with the desire for individuality and autonomy. One is tempted to suggest that totally free, autonomous, and personal decisions about what kind of a hospital to build, where, and for whom are increasingly incompatible with equitable and efficient delivery of services to all the people. We live in a society which gives high priority to free enterprise and resistance to government controls; but the widespread desire for better medical care compels the development of rationally planned facilities which are located, staffed, and operated with the best interests of the population at large in mind. It is commonplace to assert that such broad social interests may not always coincide with the perceived interests of groups whose right of decision may be pre-empted.

The Heart, Cancer, and Stroke legislation[5] of 1965 may turn out to be the most influential single factor to date in setting up comprehensive regional medical programs. One suspects, however, that the selection of these particular diseases was based upon political rather than medical or organizational factors and that the term "related diseases" was added presumably as a result of pressures brought to bear by agents and agencies which would otherwise be "dealt out" of this first massive medical system reorganization.[6]

Ultimately, of course, reorganization of *any* kind is bound to have some effects on existing medical systems. A major question is whether actually building new medical bricks-and-mortar to treat special disease entities will help or hinder the over-all organization of a total health care system. The alternative is to go along with the existing facilities and attempt to enhance their effectiveness and collaborative potential as much as possible. The express care with which local autonomy is being handled is at once salutory and dangerous. The implicit danger in this approach is the persistence of old forms with limited utility together with the addition of new forms that *may* prove to be expensive, overly specific, and difficult to dislodge even when demonstrated to be undesirable.

THE OLD PROBLEMS AND THE "NEW LOOK"

One important outcome of this desire for comprehensive and efficient medical care is that it helps to create an awareness of the glaring defiencies in knowledge and techniques of care which must be overcome. We do not have in mind those well-defined and well-understood conditions for which there is no known cure, but those where the technology for treatment or prevention is known but underutilized. For example, mental health remains an intractable conundrum and a barely assessable complicator of all kinds of health problems. In general, the therapies used for mental and emotional illness comprise the least well-defined and organized body of knowledge in medicine. Much of it, indeed, lies outside the formal boundaries of medicine. It is precisely in the area of mental health that it is most difficult to enlist the aid of ill people in their own behalf, even when physical, financial, and professional barriers have largely been removed. It remains true that there are many ways in which mental health services can be offered which themselves mitigate against full successful utilization. So it appears that as the hospital or system expands to include more and more of the total patient, the system and the patient himself may actually obstruct and hinder the healing process.

In the Montefiore demonstration, for example, it turned out that the mere availability of a social worker on the health team did not result in automatic acceptance of her services. The discovery of psychiatric problems and the offer of referral (with payment not an issue) did not always result in acceptance by the patient either. It is exactly at this coming together of the patient and the agents of the medical system that it is most difficult to fix responsibility for lack of utilization: Is it the intractable and unimaginative organizational system or only the recalcitrant patient?

Health education and preventive medicine also turn out to be areas in which more is required than just the willingness of professionals to entertain novel ideas and the availability of funds. For example, a Philadelphia hospital set out to implement those aspects of comprehensive care which pertain to preventive measures *and* to education for positive health.

To do this many radical departures from ordinary hospital practices were made.[7] The authors concluded their report with a plea to sociology to supply them with the tools to do the job. The hospital had the facility and the medical knowledge; what was lacking was a conceptual basis both to inform the reorganization and to evaluate it.

While much of the above seems to forebode dissappointment, there are some positive aspects which now ought to be mentioned. In fact, what we are beginning to "know for sure" (in some cases with well-organized supporting data) is by no means negligible.

The "New" Hospital. Hospitals can redefine their roles, reorganize their patterns of work, and still survive. In many of the cases cited in this book there was some degree of success in adopting more comprehensive definitions of patient care and in softening the hard impact of impersonal "bureaucratic" modalities. There seems to be little question that broad and long-term oriented action in health *can* result from hospitals having altered their boundaries, internal structure, and external relationships. Certain of the components of the "new" hospital most commonly reported are improved staff-patient relationships, moving staff teams into closer and more continuous contact with particular patient groups, and a splitting-off of certain patient needs from others in order to use scarce resources more judiciously and to meet more nearly the requirements of personalized care.

The "New" Patient. At least on paper, the patient is coming into his own right as the owner and interpreter of his symptoms, his attitudes toward health and medicine, and his preferences for types of care. Perhaps more important, he is increasingly coming to be regarded as the co-author of the outcome of any treatment program. More than ever before, the patient is being solicited as an active participant in the pursuit of positive health. And a galaxy of changes in medical care are in the making once the patient is no longer regarded as a passive recipient of medicines, manipulations, and prescriptions.

The "New" Doctor. The general practitioner, as he once was, has all but disappeared. We may not be certain just who will fill the role, but there is some basis for speculating about the qualities and attributes he will need to have. First, he will probably still have to bear the title "Doctor," whoever he turns out to be, for it appears that most patients will accept only this for now.[8] At the same time, the specialist and research scientist in medicine are certainly going to be indispensable if only because they provide the solid procedural base of medical knowledge and practice.

One might speculate that the modern doctor of the future will have to combine aspects of *both* the general practitioner *and* the specialist. Just as the hospital of the future is likely to try to address and respond to *both* the humanistic and technical themes in contemporary society, so too medicine's representatives, personified in the physician, will be called upon to orient themselves toward their patients in *both* these ways. There are some signs that students in medical schools are showing heightened awareness of the need to practice general medicine at the same time as they reject the traditional role of the "g.p." To this end, a medical student newsletter endorsed the recommendations of the Millis report which calls for the development of a *scientific* way of meeting *human* needs that will not make the persons being treated something less than human.

Whether we can have it *all* ways at once—humanely responsive and technologically sharp; specific and broad; crisis-oriented and long-term; lateral *and* nonlateral; longitudinal *and* nonlongitudinal—is perhaps the key question for the future hospital and for those who shall fall ill.

Notes

Chapter 1

1. U.S. Department of Health, Education and Welfare, *Vital and Health Statistics*, "Personal Health Expenses," Washington, D.C., Series 10, No. 22, 1965, p. 2.
2. *Ibid.*, "Physician Visits—Health Statistics," Series 10, No. 18, June 1965.
3. *Ibid.*, "Chronic Conditions Causing Limitation of Activities," Series B, No. 36, October 1962.
4. *Ibid.*, "Utilization of Institutions for the Aged and Chronically Ill," Series 12, No. 4, February 1966.
5. *Ibid.*, "Hospitalization in the Last Year of Life," Series 22, No. 1, September 1965.
6. *Ibid.*
7. Oswald Hall, "The Changing Public Image of the Changing Hospital," *Hospital Administration*, 9 (Fall 1964), 6–14.
8. William R. Rosengren, "Communication, Organization, and Conduct in the Therapeutic Milieu," *Administrative Science Quarterly*, 9 (June 1964), 70–90.
9. Warren Bennis, *Changing Organizations*, New York, McGraw-Hill, 1966.
10. Harold K. Wilensky and C. N. Lebeaux, *Industrial Society and Social Welfare*, New York, The Free Press, 1965, p. vii.
11. *Ibid.*
12. Robert N. Wilson, "Physicians' Changing Hospital Role," *Human Organization*, 18 (Winter 1959–1960), 177–183.
13. The manner by which order and structure in hospitals is achieved through interaction rather than fashioned in advance is set forth in Anselm Strauss, et al., "The Hospital and its Negotiated Order," in *The Hospital in Modern Society*, E. Freidson, ed, New York, The Free Press, 1963.

Chapter 2

1. "Shaping the Health Care Revolution," *Medical World News*, 8:34 (August 25, 1967), 56–65.
2. E. R. Weinerman, "Anchor Points Underlying the Planning for Tomorrow's Health Care," *Bulletin of the New York Academy of Medicine*, 41 (December 1965), 1213–1226.

3. Department of Hospitals and Medical Facilities, "The Emergency Department: Problem and Overview," *Journal of the American Medical Association,* 198: 4 (1966), 380–383.

4. E. R. Weinerman, R. S. Ratner, A. Robbins, and M. Lavenhar, "Yale Studies in Ambulatory Medical Care: Determinants of Use of Hospital E. R.," *American Journal of Public Health,* 56:7 (1966), 1037–1056.

5. Ward Darley and Anne R. Somers, "Medicine, Money, and Manpower: The Challenge to Professional Education," *The New England Journal of Medicine,* 276 (June 22, 1967), 1414–1422.

6. George A. Silver, "Social Medicine at the Montefiore Hospital: A Practical Approach to Community Health Problems," *American Journal of Public Health,* 48 (June 1958), 724–731.

7. George A. Silver, *Family Medical Care,* Cambridge, Harvard University Press, 1963.

8. George A. Silver, "Social Medicine at the Montefiore Hospital," *op. cit.,* 724–731.

9. Eliot Freidson, *Patients' Views of Medical Practice,* New York, The Russell Sage Foundation, 1961.

10. J. C. Matchar, F. F. Furstenberg, and H. P. Kalisch, "Comprehensive Medical Care: Sinai Hospital's Approach to Medical Care for the Aged," *Gerontologist,* 5:3 (1965), 125–128.

11. *Ibid.,* p. 126.

12. P. Rogatz and G.M. Crocetti, "Home Care Programs: Their Impact on the Hospital's Role in Medical Care," *American Journal of Public Health,* 48 (September 1958), 1125–1133.

13. William Hubbard, quoted in " 'Health Complex' Seen Superseding Present Hospital," *Medical News* (May 15, 1967).

14. J. S. Beloff and E. R. Weinerman, "Yale Studies in Family Health Care: Planning and Pilot Test of a New Program," *Journal of the American Medical Association,* 199 (February 6, 1967), 383–389.

15. I. H. Strantz and W. R. Miller, "Development of Interagency Coordination in a Program of Comprehensive Medical Care," *American Journal of Public Health,* 56 (May 1966), 785–796.

16. *Ibid.,* p. 795.

17. J. E. Garland, *An Experiment in Medicine: The First Twenty Years of the Pratt Clinic and the New England Center Hospital of Boston,* Cambridge, The Riverside Press, 1960.

18. Ray E. Trussell. *Hunterdon Medical Center: The Story of One Approach to Rural Medical Care,* Cambridge, Published for the Commonwealth Fund by Harvard University Press, 1956.

19. W. J. McNerney and D. C. Riedel, *Regionalization and Rural Health Care: An Experiment in Three Communities,* Ann Arbor, University of Michigan Graduate School of Business Administration, Research Series No. 2, 1962.

Chapter 3

1. The importance of this has been stressed in terms of both empirical statements and quite abstract formulations. Peter M. Blau, "Orientations Toward Clients in a Public Welfare Agency," *Administrative Science Quarterly*, 5 (December 1960), 245–261; Amitai Etzioni, *A Comparative Analysis of Complex Organizations*, New York, The Free Press, 1961, are representative of each type.

2. For example, Michel Crozier, *The Bureaucratic Phenomenon*, Chicago, University of Chicago Press, 1964; Eugene Haas, R. Hall, and N. Johnson, "The Size of Supportive Components in Organizations," *Social Forces*, 42 (October 1963), 9–17; Robert Merton, "Bureaucratic Structure and Personality," in *Social Theory and Social Structure*, New York, The Free Press, 1949, 151–160; Arthur Stinchcombe, "Bureaucratic and Craft Administration of Production," *Administrative Science Quarterly*, 4 (September 1959), 168–187; Stanley Udy, Jr., "Bureaucratic Elements in Organizations: Some Research Findings," *American Sociological Review*, 23 (August 1958), 415–418.

3. A.M. Henderson and Talcott Parsons, trans. and eds., *Max Weber: The Theory of Social and Economic Organization*, New York, Oxford University Press, 1947.

4. See, for example, Mary E. W. Goss, "Influence and Authority Among Physicians in an Out-Patient Clinic," *American Sociological Review*, 26 (February 1961), 39–50; David Solomon, "Professional Persons in Bureaucratic Organizations," in *Symposium on Preventive and Social Psychiatry*, Washington, Walter Reed Army Institute, 1958, 253–266; Eugene Litwak, "Models of Bureaucracy Which Permit Conflict," *American Journal of Sociology*, 67 (September 1961), 177–184.

5. Charles Perrow, "Hospitals: Technology, Structure, and Goals," in *Handbook of Organizations*, James March, ed., Chicago, Rand McNally, 1965, p. 959.

6. *Ibid.*

7. William R. Rosengren, "Structure, Policy, and Style: Strategies of Organizational Control," *Administrative Science Quarterly*, 12 (June 1967), 140–164.

8. William Glaser, "American and Foreign Hospitals," in *The Hospital in Modern Society*, E. Freidson, ed., New York, The Free Press, 1963, 37–42.

9. Charles Perrow, "The Analysis of Goals in Complex Organizations," *American Sociological Review*, 26 (December 1961), 854–866.

10. Charles Perrow, "Goals and Power Structures—A Historical Case Study," in *The Hospital in Modern Society, op. cit.*, 112–146.

11. Eliot Freidson and Buford Rhea, "Processes of Control in a Company of Equals," *Social Problems*, 11 (Fall 1963), 119–131.
12. W. Glaser, *op. cit.*
13. William Caudill, "Around the Clock Patient Care in Japanese Psychiatric Hospitals: The Role of the *Tsukisoi*," *American Sociological Review*, 26 (April 1961), 204–214.
14. Rose L. Coser, "Authority and Decision-Making in a Hospital," *American Sociological Review*, 23 (February 1958), 56–63.
15. Melvin Seeman and J. Evans, "Stratification and Hospital Care: I. The Performance of the Medical Interne," *American Sociological Review*, 26 (February 1961), 67–80.
16. *Ibid.*
17. Peter M. Blau, *Bureaucracy in Modern Society*, New York, Random House, 1956, p. 34.
18. Alfred H. Stanton and Morris S. Schwartz, *The Mental Hospital*, New York, Basic Books, 1954.
19. Athan Karras, Sister Joan Marie Upjohn, and Mark Lefton, "Methodological and Practical Considerations for Studying the Effects of Change in Ward Administration On Staff and Patients," *Comprehensive Psychiatry*, 4 (October 1963), 343–350.
20. Mark Lefton, Simon Dinitz, and Benjamin Pasamanick, "Decision-Making in a Mental Hospital: Real, Perceived, and Ideal," *American Sociological Review*, 24 (December 1959), 822–829.

Chapter 4

1. Rose L. Coser, *Life on the Ward*, East Lansing, Michigan State University Press, 1962.
2. *Ibid.*
3. *Ibid.*, p. 46.
4. Amitai Etzioni, *A Comparative Analysis of Complex Organizations*, New York, The Free Press, 1961.
5. *Ibid.*
6. *Ibid.*, p. 50.
7. Renée Fox, *Experiment Perilous*, New York, The Free Press, 1959.
8. The expectation to "get well" is regarded as central to the normative conduct of ill persons. But Talcott Parsons' now classic discussion of the "sick role" seems to be most relevant to those illnesses in which the probability of *actually* "getting well" is objectively present.
9. A parallel perspective informs the one major study of medical education which represents the symbolic interaction and conflict tradition, Howard S. Becker, et al., *Boys in White*, Chicago, University of Chicago Press, 1961.
10. Julius A. Roth, *Timetables*, Indianapolis, Bobbs-Merrill, 1963.

11. William R. Rosengren, "A Longitudinal View of Patient Conduct," *Journal of Nervous and Mental Disease*, 137 (November 1963), 466–478.

12. Bruno Bettelheim, *The Empty Fortress*, New York, The Free Press, 1967.

13. The importance of differing organizational definitions of patient materials has been stressed by Eliot Freidson, "Disability as Social Deviance," in *Sociology and Rehabilitation*, M. B. Sussman, ed., Washington, Vocational Rehabilitation Administration, 1966; Mark Lefton and William R. Rosengren, "Organizations and Clients: Lateral and Longitudinal Dimensions," *American Sociological Review*, 31 (December 1966), 802–810; Charles Perrow, "A Framework for the Comparative Analysis of Organizations, "*American Sociological Review*, 31 (April 1967), 194–208.

14. Albert F. Wessen, "The Apparatus of Rehabilitation," in *Sociology and Rehabilitation, op. cit.*

15. B. Glaser and A. Strauss, *Awareness of Dying*, Chicago, Aldine, 1965.

16. A clear statement of the changing character of rules and rule-making in hospitals is found in Anselm Strauss, et al., "The Hospital and its Negotiated Order," in *The Hospital in Modern Society*, E. Friedson, ed., New York, The Free Press, 1963.

17. W. Glaser and A. Strauss, *Awareness of Dying, op. cit.*, p. 15.

18. A. Strauss, et al., "The Hospital and its Negotiated Order," in *The Hospital in Modern Society, op. cit.*, p. 153.

19. *Ibid.*

20. See the discussion in Jules Henry, "The Formal Social Structure of a Psychiatric Hospital," in *Sociological Studies of Health and Illness*, D. Apple, ed., New York, McGraw-Hill, 1960, 260–279.

21. Erving Goffman, *Asylums*, New York, Doubleday Anchor, 1961.

22. *Ibid.*, x.

23. William Caudill, review of Erving Goffman's *Asylums, in American Journal of Sociology*, 68 (November 1962), 336–369.

24. Ivan Belknap, *The Human Problems of a State Mental Hospital*, New York, McGraw-Hill, 1956; H. Warren Dunham and S. Kirson Weinberg, *The Culture of the State Mental Hospital*, Detroit, Wayne State University Press, 1960.

25. This is a point much discussed between Rosengren and Harold W. Pfautz of Brown University. Professor Pfautz to whose insight we are indebted, likens institutions of this character to expressive social movements.

26. Charles Perrow has also stressed this pattern in "Hospitals: Technology, Structure, and Goals," in *Handbook of Organizations*, James March, ed., Chicago, Rand McNally, 1965, 910–971.

27. J. Sanbourne Bockoven, *Moral Treatment in American Psychiatry*, New York, Springer, 1963.
28. *Ibid.*, p. 19.
29. William Caudill, *The Psychiatric Hospital as a Small Society*, Cambridge, Harvard University Press, 1958.
30. Robert W. Hyde, et al., *Milieu Rehabilitation*. Providence, Butler Health Center, 1962. p. 27.
31. See especially Robert Rapoport, Rhona Rapoport, and I. Rosow, *Community as Doctor*, London, Tavistock, 1960.
32. This has been discussed as "psuedo-democracy" in Peter M. Blau and W. Richard Scott, *Formal Organizations*, San Francisco, Chandler, 1962.
33. M. Lefton, S. Dinitz, and B. Pasamanick, "Decision-Making a Mental Hospital: Real, Perceived, and Ideal, "*American Sociological Review*, 24 (December 1959), 822–829.
34. This is parallel to processes which occur in some schools and universities. See, for example, Charles E. Bidwell and Rebecca Vreeland, "College Education and Moral Orientations," *Administrative Science Quarterly*, 8 (September 1963), 166–191.
35. See for example Charles Perrow, "A Framework for the Comparative Analysis of Formal Organizations," *American Sociological Review*, 26 (1967), 104–208.
36. *Ibid.*
37. W. R. Rosengren and S. DeVault, "The Sociology of Time and Space in an Obstetrical Hospital," in *The Hospital in Modern Society, op. cit.*, 283.
38. This is a point very heavily emphasized by Perrow, "A Framework for the Comparative Analysis of Formal Organizations," *op. cit.*
39. James D. Thompson, *Organizations in Action*. New York, McGraw-Hill, 1967.
40. Selwyn W. Becker and Gerald Gordon, "An Entrepreneurial Theory of Formal Organizations. Part I: Patterns of Formal Organizations, *Administrative Science Quarterly*, 11 (September 1966), 315–344.
41. Eliot Freidson, "Disability as Social Deviance," in *Sociology and Rehabilitation, op. cit.*, 71–99.

Chapter 5

1. Sol Levine and Paul E. White, "The Community of Health Organizations," in *Handbook of Medical Sociology*. Howard E. Freeman, Sol Levine, and Leo G. Reader, eds., Englewood Cliffs, Prentice-Hall, 1963.
2. *Ibid.*, p. 321.
3. J. Sanbourne Bockoven, *Moral Treatment in American Psychiatry*, *op. cit.*

4. Ivan Belknap and John Steinle, *The Community and Its Hospitals,* Syracuse, Syracuse University Press, 1963.

5. Harold W. Pfautz and Gita Wilder, "The Ecology of a Mental Hospital," *Journal of Health and Human Behavior,* 3 (Summer 1962), 67–72.

6. L. Vaughn Blankenship and Ray Elling, "Organizational Support and Community Power Structure," *Journal of Health and Human Behavior,* 3 (Winter 1962), 257–269.

7. *Ibid.,* p. 268.

8. Charles Perrow, "Goals and Power Structures—A Historical Case Study, in *The Hospital in Modern Society,* E. Freidson, ed., New York, The Free Press, 1963, 112–146.

9. Eliot Freidson, *Patients' Views of Medical Practice,* New York, The Russell Sage Foundation, 1961.

10. *Ibid.,* p. 145.

11. Eliot Freidson, "Specialities Without Roots," *Human Organization,* 18 (Fall 1959), 112–116; Reprinted in W. Richard Scott and Edmund Volkart, eds., *Medical Care, Readings in the Sociology of Medical Institutions,* New York, Wiley, 1966, p. 448.

12. Oswald Hall, "The Informal Organization of Medical Practice," *Canadian Journal of Economics and Political Science,* 12:2 (1946), 30–44; O. Hall, "The Stages of a Medical Career, *American Journal of Sociology,* 53 (March 1948), 327–336.

13. Stanley Lieberson, "Ethnic Groups and the Practice of Medicine," *American Sociological Review,* 23 (October 1958), 542–549.

14. *Ibid.*

15. *Ibid.*

16. David N. Solomon, "Ethnic and Class Differences Among Hospitals as Contingencies in Medical Careers," *American Journal of Sociology,* 66 (March 1961), 463–471.

17. C. Perrow, "Goals and Power Structures," *op. cit.,* 112–146.

18. Eugene Litwak and L. Hylton, "Interorganizational Analysis," *Administrative Science Quarterly,* 6 (March 1962), 395–420.

19. *Ibid.,* p. 396.

20. William Evan, "The Organizational Set: Toward a Theory of Interorganizational Relations," in *Organizational Design,* James D. Thompson, ed., Pittsburgh University of Pittsburgh Press, 1966.

21. *Ibid.,* p. 175.

22. Albert Wessen, "The Apparatus of Rehabilitation" in *Sociology and Rehabilitation,* M. B. Sussman, ed., Washington, Vocational Rehabilitation Administration, 1966, p. 153.

23. *Ibid.,* p. 164.

24. *Ibid.*

25. Ray Elling, "The Hospital Support Game in Urban Center," in *The Hospital in Modern Society, op. cit.,* 73–111.

26. Sol Levine and Paul White, "Exchange as a Conceptual Framework for the study of Interorganizational Relationships," *Administrative Science Quarterly*, 5 (March 1961), 585.
27. James D. Thompson and William J. McEwen, "Organizational Goals and Environment: Goal-Setting as an Interaction Process," *American Sociological Review*, 23 (February 1958), 23–31.
28. *Ibid.*, p. 30.
29. William Evan, "The Organizational Set," *op. cit.*, 173–191.
30. *Ibid.*, p. 179.
31. *Ibid.*, p. 181.
32. Sol Levine and Paul White, "Exchange as a Conceptual Framework for the Study of Interorganizational Relations," *op. cit.*, p. 597.

Chapter 6

1. Talcott Parsons, "Suggestions for a Sociological Approach to the Theory of Organizations," in A. Etzioni, ed., *Complex Organizations: A Sociological Reader*, New York, Holt, Rinehart and Winston, 1961, 39–40.
2. Peter Blau and W. R. Scott, *Formal Organizations*, San Francisco: Chandler, 1962, p. 77.
3. Charles Perrow, "Hospitals; Technology, Structure, and Goals," in *Handbook of Organizations*, James March, ed., Chicago, Rand McNally, 1965, 650–677.
4. Amitai Etzioni, *Modern Organizations*. Englewood Cliffs, Prentice-Hall, 1964, p. 94.
5. S. N. Eisenstadt, "Bureaucracy, Bureaucratization, and De bureaucratization," in A. Etzioni, *Complex Organizations: A Sociological Reader*, *op. cit.*, p. 276.
6. W. Glaser and A. Strauss, *Awareness of Dying*, Chicago, Aldine, 1965, 284.
7. Everett C. Hughes, *Men and Their Work*, New York, The Free Press, 1958, p. 11, *passim*.
8. An aspect of clients in organizations pursued in the next chapter has to do with the content of the socialization process and its effects upon the patient. One issue here has to do with the consequences of socialization for behavior expectations on the one hand and for the internalization of values on the other. See, for example, Robert Dubin, "Deviant Behavior and Social Structure," *American Sociological Review*, 24 (April 1959), 147–164; Irving Rosow, "Forms and Functions of Adult Socialization," *Social Forces*, 44 (September 1965), 35–45.
9. William R. Rosengren, "Longitudinal View of Patient Conduct," *Journal of Nervous and Mental Disease*, 137 (November 1963), 467.
10. See for example, Rose Laub Coser, "Laughter Among Colleagues,"

Psychiatry, 23 (February 1960), 81–95; Robert N. Wilson, "Teamwork in the Operating Room," *Human Organization*, 12 (Winter 1954), 9–14; Julius Roth, "Ritual and Magic in the Control of Contagion," *American Sociological Review*, 22 (June 1957), 310–314; William R. Rosengren and Spencer DeVault, "The Sociology of Time and Space in an Obstetrical Hospital," in *The Hospital in Modern Society*, E. Friedson, ed., New York, The Free Press, 1963, 266–292.

11. Bernard M. Kramer, *Day Hospital*, New York, Grune & Stratton, 1962, p. 66.

12. Anselm Strauss, et al., "The Hospital and Its Negotiated Order," in *The Hospital in Modern Society, op. cit.*

13. These processes have been described in the now extensive literature in social psychiatry dealing with "milieu therapy" institutions. See for example, Milton Greenblatt, R. York, and E. Brown, *From Custodial to Therapeutic Patient Care in Psychiatric Hospitals*, New York, Russell Sage Foundation, 1955; Mark Lefton, S. Dinitz, and B. Pasamanick, "Decision-Making in a Mental Hospital: Real, Perceived, and Ideal," *American Sociological Review*, 24 (December 1959), 822–829; Robert Rapoport and Rhona Rapoport, "Democratization and Authority in a Therapeutic Community," *Behavioral Sciences*, 2 (April 1957), 128–133; William R. Rosengren, "Communication, Organization, and Conduct in the 'Therapeutic Milieu,'" *Administrative Science Quarterly*, 9 (June 1964), 70–90.

14. Some implications of the pine- and oak-tree structures are set forth in Jules Henry, "The Formal Social Structure of a Psychiatric Hospital," in *Sociological Studies of Health and Sickness*, D. Apple, ed., New York, McGraw-Hill, 1960, 260–279.

15. Rose L. Coser, *Life on the Ward*, East Lansing, Michigan State University Press, 1962, p. 15.

16. J. Henry, "The Formal Social Structure of a Psychiatric Hospital," *op. cit.*, p. 265.

17. R. L. Coser, *Life on the Ward, op. cit.*, 133–134.

18. J. Henry, "The Formal Social Structure of a Psychiatric Hospital," *op. cit.*, 265.

19. William R. Rosengren, "Organizational Age, Structure, and Orientation Toward Clients," *Social Forces*, 47 (September 1968), 1–11.

20. Reference is to the distinction between the "local," whose identity and commitment is to a specific organization, and the "cosmopolitan" who identifies more generally with his professional network. For example, it was found that the "locally" oriented medical sociologist worked in debureaucratized (broadly oriented) hospitals, while "cosmopolitans" worked in bureaucratic (specifically focused) organizations: William R. Rosengren, "Sociologists in Medicine: Organizational Contexts and Professional Careers," in *The Professional*

in the Organization, M. Abrahamson, ed., Chicago, Rand McNally, 1967, 143–155.

21. See David Mechanic, "Sources of Power of Lower Participants in Complex Organizations," *Administrative Science Quarterly,* 7 (December 1962), 349–364.

22. W. Rosengren, "Communication, Organization, and Conduct in the Therapeutic Milieu," *Administrative Science Quarterly,* 9 (June 1964), 85.

23. Robert W. Hyde, et al., *Milieu Rehabilitation,* Providence, Butler Health Center, 1962, p. 27.

24. This kind of "assembly-line" technology has been called "long-linked," James D. Thompson, *Organizations in Action,* New York, McGraw-Hill, 1967.

25. W. R. Rosengren and S. DeVault, "The Sociology of Time and Space in an Obstetrical Hospital, in *The Hospital in Modern Society, op. cit.,* p. 283.

26. David Mechanic, *Medical Sociology: A Selective View,* New York, The Free Press, 1968, p. 88.

27. W. R. Rosengren and S. DeVault, "The Sociology of Time and Space . . . ," *op. cit.,* p. 282.

28. B. Kramer, *Day Hospital, op cit.,* 40–41.

29. The importance of interpersonal relationships not strictly medical in nature have often been regarded as especially salient in hospitals of this type, see Alfred H. Stanton and Morris S. Schwartz, *The Mental Hospital,* New York, Basic Books, 1954; William Caudill, *The Psychiatric Hospital as a Small Society,* Cambridge, Harvard University Press and the Commonwealth Fund, 1958.

Chapter 7

1. I. Rosow, "Forms and Functions of Adult Socialization," *Social Forces,* 44 (September 1965), 35–45.

2. Some of the ways in which treatment ideologies can be turned to deal with organizational problems are discussed in W. R. Rosengren, "Communication, Organization, and Conduct in the Therapeutic Milieu," *Administrative Science Quarterly,* 9 (June 1964), 70–90.

3. P. Blau and W. R. Scott, *Formal Organizations,* San Francisco, Chandler, 1962, p. 188.

4. C. Perrow, "Hospitals: Technology, Structure, and Goals, in *Handbook of Organizations,* James March, ed., Chicago, Rand McNally, 1965.

5. David Landy and Milton Greenblatt, *Halfway House,* Washington, Vocational Rehabilitation Administration, 1965, 87, *passim.*

6. Orville G. Brim, Jr., and Stanton Wheeler, *Socialization After Childhood,* New York, Wiley, 1965, p. 60.

7. William R. Rosengren, "Social Class and Becoming 'Ill,'" in *Blue-Collar World*, A. Shostak and W. Gomberg, eds., Englewood Cliffs, Prentice-Hall 1964, p. 339.

8. Frances P. MacGregor, "Some Psycho-Social Problems Associated with Facial Deformities," in *Patients, Physicians, and Illness*, E. G. Jaco, ed., New York, The Free Press, 1958, p. 276.

9. D. Landy and M. Greenblatt, *Halfway House, op. cit.*, p. 93.

10. O. G. Brim, Jr., and S. Wheeler, *Socialization After Childhood, op. cit.*, 62–63.

11. Erving Goffman, "On the Characteristics of Total Institutions," in *The Prison*, D. Cressey, ed., New York, Holt, Rinehart and Winston, 1961, p. 24.

12. J. Roth, *Timetables*, Indianapolis, Bobbs-Merrill, 1963, p. 102.

13. See Fred Davis, "Uncertainty in Medical Prognosis: Clinical and Functional," *American Journal of Sociology*, 66 (July 1960), 41–47.

14. Clark E. Moustakas, *Loneliness*, Englewood Cliffs, Prentice-Hall, 1961, p. xiii.

15. *Ibid.*

16. W. R. Rosengen and S. DeVault, "The Sociology of Time and Space in an Obstetrical Hospital," *op. cit.*, in *Hospital in Modern Society*, E. Freidson, ed., New York, The Free Press, 1963.

17. Milton Davis and Robert von der Lippe, "Discharge From Hospital Against Medical Advice," presented at the meetings of the American Sociological Association, Chicago, August 1965 (mimeographed).

18. H. Warren Dunham and S. Kirson Weinberg, *The Culture of the State Mental Hospital*, Detroit, Wayne State University Press, 1960, p. 71.

19. *Ibid.*, p. 68.

20. *Ibid.*, p. 76.

21. *Ibid.*, p. 82.

22. Fred Davis, *Passage Through Crisis*, Indianapolis, Bobbs-Merrill, 1963, p. 79.

23. *Ibid.*, p. 69. *passim.*

24. J. Roth, *Timetables, op. cit.*, p. 41.

25. B. Glaser and A. Strauss, *Awareness of Dying*, Chicago, Aldine, 1965, p. 80.

26. *Ibid.*

27. Thomas Scheff, "Typification in the Diagnostic Practices of Rehabilitation Agencies," in *Sociology and Rehabilitation*, M. B. Sussman, ed., Washington, Vocational Rehabilitation Administration, 1966, p. 139, *passim.*

28. E. Goffman, *Stigma*, Englewood Cliffs, Prentice-Hall, 1963, p. 136.

29. W. R. Rosengren and S. DeVault, "The Sociology of Time and Space . . . ," *op. cit.*, p. 290.

30. R. W. Hyde, et al., *Milieu Rehabilitation*, Providence Butler Health Center, 1962, p. 31.
31. R. A. Scott, "Comments About Interpersonal Processes of Rehabilitation," *op. cit.*, p. 138.
32. E. Goffman, *Stigma*, *op. cit.*, p. 35.
33. Robert Edgerton, *The Cloak of Competence*, Berkeley, University of California Press, 1967, 215–216.
34. *Ibid.*, p. 145.

Chapter 8

1. Public Law 89–749.
2. *Ibid.*, p. 2.
3. *Ibid.*, p. 3.
4. See for example Charles V. Willie and Herbert Notkin, "Community Organization for Health: A Case Study," in *Patients, Physicians and Illness*, E. Gartly Jaco, ed., New York, The Free Press, 1958.
5. J. H. Robb, "Family Structure and Agency Coordination: Decentralisation and the Citizen," in *Social Welfare Institutions*, Mayer N. Zald, ed., New York, Wiley, 1965, p. 393.
6. Large-scale clinical "follow-up" investigations of the outcomes of treatment is one way—perhaps often unintended—by which hospitals may extend their interests in patients over time.
7. William R. Rosengren, "Organizational Age, Structure, and Orientations Toward Clients," *Social Forces*, 47 (September 1968), 1–11.
8. See R. E. Trussell, *Hunterdon Medical Center*; W. J. McNerney and D. C. Riedel, *Regionalization and Rural Health Care*, *op. cit.*
9. Special economic interests and arrangements, especially the incentives involved in maintaining higher levels of worker health as a result of lowered insurance rates, sometimes bring such transformation of goals and organizations.
10. See George A. Silver, "Social Medicine at the Montefiore Hospital: A Practical Approach to Community Health Problems," *American Journal of Public Health*, 48 (June 1958), 724–731.
11. See for example the several accounts in *Community Action Against Poverty*, George A. Brager and Francis P. Purcell, eds., New Haven, College and University Press, 1967.
12. Much of this discussion is drawn from Mark Lefton, "The Role of the Counsellor and Agency Structure." Unpublished manuscript.
13. Albert Wessen, "The Apparatus of Rehabilitation," in *Sociology and Rehabilitation*, M. B. Sussman, ed., Washington, Vocational Rehabilitation Administration, 1966, p. 153.
14. *Medical Care: Readings in the Sociology of Medical Institutions*,

W. Richard Scott and Edmund Volkart, eds., New York, Wiley, 1966, p. 1.

15. This kind of concern is consistent with the development of preventive medicine programs to the degree that "longitudinality" of orientation may be thought of as extending "backward" in time as well as "forward."

16. See Chapter 6 for a discussion of this issue.

17. Warren Hagstrom, "The Power of the Poor," in *Mental Health of the Poor*, Frank Riessman, Jerome Cohen, and Arthur Pearl, eds., New York, The Free Press, 1964, 205–223.

18. Gideon Sjoberg, "Bureaucracy and the Lower Class," *Sociology and Social Research*, 50 (April 1966), 330–331.

Epilogue

1. National Commission on Community Health Services, *Health Care Facilities—The Community Bridge to Effective Health Services*. Washington, D.C., Public Affairs Press, 1963.

2. *Conference on Regional Medical Programs: Proceedings*, U.S. Department of Health, Education and Welfare, Division of Regional Medical Programs, Washington, D.C., U.S. 1967, p. 111.

3. S. Farber, *Ibid.*, p. 28.

4. "Better Neighborhood Health Centers are Sought for Poor in Urban Areas," *Medical News*, February 27, 1967.

5. Public Law 89–239, October 6, 1965.

6. J. M. Russell, "New Federal Regional Medical Programs," *The New England Journal of Medicine*, 275 (August 11, 1966), 309–312.

7. K. E. Langwill and E. H. Vick, "Lankenau Hospital's Community Health Education Program," *American Journal of Public Health*, 48 (November 1958), 1507–1511.

8. Eliot Freidson, in G. A. Silver, "Social Medicine at the Montefiore Hospital: A Practical Approach to Community Health Problems," *American Journal of Public Health*, 48 (June 1958), 212.

Name Index

Subject Index

Aged, and Sinai Hospital, Baltimore, 25, 27–28

Bureaucratic structure of hospital
conflict in mental hospitals, 66–67
control styles: patient and personnel, 57–60
division of labor, 57
and medical ward, 61–63
modes of patient care, 57–58
and physician hierarchy, 55–56, 63–64
relationship to technology, 57–59, 63
supervisory style, 57
and surgical ward, 61–63

Chronically ill, and Montefiore Hospital experiment, New York, 25–26
Comprehensive care, role of the hospital in, 19, 25–27, 34

Death
and medical organization setting, 10, 160
and the patient, 80–81, 160–161
Disease
and cancer ward, 80–81
changes in concept of, 20
changes in patterns of, 20
incurable, 76–77
tuberculosis, 77–78

Emergency room
increased use of, 22
as indicator of stress, 21
as medical resource for low-income groups, 22

Formal organizations
focus on client patient, 5
and technological orientation, 5–6

Health complexes
as core facility, 31–32
as differentiated from the medical center, 32–33
organization of, 31, 32
as patient-centered, 31–32
Home care services
Aging Center, Sinai Hospital, 25, 27, 28, 30
contribution to medical education, 28–29
Montifiore program for chronically ill, 25–26, 30
relationship to the hospital, 27, 30
Hospitals
and the aged chronically ill, 26–28
authority structure and orientation to patient, 131–134
bureaucratic structure of, 48–68
and client biography perspective, 119–144
collaboration between
and client biography model, 169–184
formal and informal, 177, 179–180
at operating-implementing level, 177, 183, 186
at policy-administrative level, 177, 183, 186
community morphology approach to, 97–109
and community power structure, 98, 101–103, 105–107, 112
and comprehensive care, 19, 21, 25–27, 34
definition of the patient, 5, 91–92, 121
domain of, 115
expectations of patient behavior, 161–166
general, 104

LaVergne, TN USA
24 April 2010
180354LV00003B/105/P